NUCLEAR MEDICINE

A PRIMER

Editor

Harmandeep Singh

Copyright

NUCLEAR MEDICINE A PRIMER

First edition 2021

Publisher: Harmandeep Singh, Department of Nuclear Medicine, PGIMER, Sector-12, Chandigarh, INDIA-160012.

Printer: Amazon kindle direct publishing (https://kdp.amazon.com), Made in Middletown, DE, USA.

Note: Full effort has been made to omit any errors and to provide valid information according to current practice. However, as knowledge and practice are rapidly changing in medicine, it is the responsibility of the readers/physicians who rely on experience and knowledge about the patient to determine the best investigations and treatment for the patient. The information contained herein is provided "as is" and without warranty of any kind. The contributors to this book disclaim responsibility for any errors or omissions or results obtained from the use of information contained herein. The authors request the readers to report any errors to nuclearmedicineaprimer@gmail.com

Dedication

This book is dedicated to our teachers, students and the Nuclear Medicine fraternity.

Preface

Medical graduates have limited knowledge about the specialty of Nuclear Medicine, as it is not taught as a separate subject at the undergraduate level. Due to rapid advancements in Nuclear Medicine, the field is now expanding, with new departments being set up at medical teaching institutions across India and the world. Moreover, with increasing access to nuclear medicine investigations, residency trainees in clinical specialties need to know about Nuclear Medicine techniques and therapies relevant to their practice. This e-book is an attempt to fulfill this need and provide a concise reading of Nuclear Medicine to medical undergraduates, postgraduates, and new trainees in the field of Nuclear Medicine. Readers are advised to read the introductory section before moving on to topics of interest, and try to interpret the images themselves.

Dr. Harmandeep Singh MD
FANMB MICNM
Associate Professor
Department of Nuclear
Medicine Post Graduate Institute
of Medical Education &
Research Chandigarh, INDIA

Contributors

All authors are affiliated to the Department of Nuclear Medicine, Post Graduate Institute of Medical Education & Research (PGIMER), Chandigarh, India.

Prof. Anish Bhattacharya, DNB PhD *Professor & Head*

Prof. Baljinder Singh, PhD *Professor*

Dr. Ashwani Sood, DNB *Additional Professor*

Dr. Jaya Shukla, PhD *Additional Professor*

Dr. Rajender Kumar, MD *Associate Professor*

Dr. Harmandeep Singh, MD *Associate Professor*

Dr. Harpreet Singh, MD *Assistant Professor*

Dr. Sunil Kumar, MD *Senior Resident*

Dr. Venkata Subramanian K, MD *Senior Resident*

Dr. Anwin Joseph K, MD *Senior Resident*

Dr. Yamini Mathur, MD *Senior Resident*

Dr. TK Nitheesh Raj, MD *Senior Resident*

Dr. Ankit Watts, PhD *Physicist*

Dr. Nivedita Rana, PhD *Physicist*

Dr. Swayamjeet S, MBBS *Junior Resident*

Dr. Karthikeyan, MBBS *Junior Resident*

Dr. Abdul Waheed, MBBS *Junior Resident*

Acknowledgements

Prof. B.R. Mittal, Prof. Anish Bhattacharya, and Prof. Baljinder Singh for their unflinching support and guidance. Prof. Anish Bhattacharya for help in designing the front cover. Dr. Venkata Subramanian K. for help in designing the basic layout of the book. All staff members and students of the department whose hard work has contributed to making this book possible.

I want to thank my wife, Dr. Rubeena Arora for being supportive and proofreading the manuscript. Gurman and Harbani for doing what they do best. My parents (S. Surinder Singh & Harminder Kaur), mother-in-law (Ajit Kaur), brother (Gagan), sisters (Suminder and Harleen), and friends for everything.

Front cover eBook logo: Designed by rawpixel.com / Freepik.

Table of Contents

Abbreviations

ADT – Androgen deprivation therapy

ALARA - As low as reasonably achievable

AR – Acute rejection

ATD – Anti thyroid drug

ATN – Acute tubular necrosis

BCC – Basal cell carcinoma

Bq – Becquerel

CAD – Coronary artery disease

CFR – Coronary flow reserve

Ci – Curie

CPPD - Calcium pyrophosphate dihydrate

CRPC - Castration-resistant prostate cancer

CSF - Cerebrospinal fluid

CT – Computed tomography

DAT – Dopamine transporter

DMSA – Dimercapto succinic acid

DSA – Digital subtraction angiography

DTPA - Diethylenetriamine pentaacetate

EC - L,L-ethylenedicysteine

ECD - Ethyl cysteinate dimer

ED – End-diastolic

EF – Ejection fraction

EHBA – Extra hepatic biliary atresia

ERNA – Equilibrium radionuclide angiography

ERPF - Effective renal plasma flow

eV – Electron volt

FBG – Fasting blood glucose

FDG - 2-Fluoro-2-deoxy-D-glucose

FET – Fluoro-ethyl tyrosine

FNH – Focal nodular hyperplasia

FTC – Follicular thyroid cancer

GBEF – Gall bladder ejection fraction

GERD – Gastroesophageal reflux disease

GET – Gastric emptying time

GFR - Glomerular filtration

rate

GHA – Glucoheptonate

GLUT – Glucose transporter

Gy – Gray

HCC – Hepatocellular carcinoma

HDN – Hydronephrosis

HMPAO - Hexamethyl propylene amine oxime

ICRP - International Commission on Radiological Protection

IDA - Imino diacetic acid

LAD – Left anterior descending

MAA - Macro-aggregated albumin

MAG3 - Mercaptoacetyltriglycine

MBF – Myocardial blood flow

MBq – Mega Becquerel

mCi – Millicurie

MDP – Methylene diphosphonate

MeV – Mega electron volt

MFR – Myocardial flow reserve

MI – Myocardial infarction

MIBG – Metaiodobenzylguanidine

MNG – Multinodular goiter

MPI – Myocardial perfusion imaging

MUGA - Multi-gated acquisition

NaF – Sodium fluoride

NCPF - Non-cirrhotic portal fibrosis

NET - Neuroendocrine tumour

NIS – Sodium-iodide symporter

PD – Peritoneal dialysis

PE – Pulmonary embolism

PET – Positron emission tomography

PFS – Progression free survival

PRRT - Peptide receptor radionuclide therapy

PSA – Prostate specific antigen

PSMA - Prostate specific membrane antigen

PTC – Papillary thyroid cancer

PUJO - Pelviureteric junction obstruction

PVNS - Pigmented villonodular synovitis

RAIU – Radioactive iodine uptake

RBC – Red blood cell

RC – Radionuclide cystography

RIGS – Radio immuno guided surgery

RIME – Radioguided intraoperative margin evaluation

RLT - Radioligand therapy

ROI – Region of interest

ROLL - Radioguided occult lesion localization

RSV – Radiosynovectomy

SC – Sulphur colloid

SCC – Squamous cell carcinoma

SIRT – Selective intra-arterial radionuclide therapy

SLNB - Sentinel lymph node biopsy

SPECT – Single photon emission computed tomography

SSA – Somatostatin analogues

SSTR - Somatostatin receptor

SUV – Standardized uptake value

TAC – Time-activity curve

TACE – Trans-arterial chemo-embolization

TFT – Thyroid function test

Tg – Thyroglobulin

TPCT – Triple phase computed tomography

TSH – Thyroid stimulating hormone

UDCA – Ursodeoxycholic acid

ULN – Upper limit of normal

μ – Micro

VQ – Ventilation perfusion

VUR – Vesicoureteral reflux

Section 1

An Introduction

Dr. Harmandeep Singh

Dr. Nivedita Rana

Dr. Ankit Watts

Prof. Baljinder Singh

1.1 What is Nuclear Medicine?

Nuclear Medicine is a branch of medicine, which deals with the administration of unsealed radiotracers to patients for diagnosis and treatment of diseases. Different radiotracers localize to specific organs using metabolic pathways, specific receptors or transporters. The administered radiotracers emit radiation, which can be imaged using highly specialized systems (like gamma camera and positron emission tomography) producing functional images, or can have therapeutic effect. Alternatively, the radioactivity can be measured within the body or in urine/blood samples to obtain clinically useful information.

In general, nuclear medicine investigations have high sensitivity. They are routinely used in oncology, infection imaging, neurology, cardiology, endocrinology, nephrology, urology, surgery, orthopedics, gastroenterology, medicine, and pulmonary medicine practice as a problem-solving tool, especially when anatomical imaging is inconclusive.

The concept of 'Theranostics' refers to the diagnosis and treatment of diseases by targeting specific metabolic pathways or receptors. The best example is radioiodine ^{131}I for diagnosis and therapy of treatment-refractory diffuse toxic goiter (Graves' disease). In addition, radionuclide therapy is also used for the treatment of metastatic cancers (thyroid, neuroendocrine tumors, neuroblastoma, prostate cancer), metastatic bone pain palliation, selective internal radiation therapy (SIRT) for liver cancer, refractory synovitis (radiosynovectomy), etc.

1.2 Radioactivity

One needs to be familiar with basic concepts of radioactivity in order to understand the subsequent sections. The fundamental particles that constitute the nucleus are neutrons and protons (together called nucleons). The stability of the nucleus is dependent upon the ratio of neutrons to protons. An unstable nucleus decays by the emission of particles like alpha (α) and beta (β^-); or energy in the form of gamma rays (γ). The spontaneous emission of radiation by the nucleus is called *radioactivity,* and the unstable nucleus is called a *radionuclide.* Each radionuclide is written as ^{A}X or X-A, where X is the chemical symbol of the element and A is the atomic mass. The conversion of the unstable nucleus to a stable nucleus is called *disintegration.* The energy of radiation emitted is measured in terms of electron volt (eV). Typical energy of radiation used in Nuclear Medicine lies in range of 10^3 (kilo) to 10^6 (Mega) electron volts. The time in which radioactivity reduces to half is called the half-life, and is characteristic of a radionuclide.

Radioactive decay is a random process, and the decay of the radioactive atom is proportional to the total number of radioactive atoms (N) present. The radioactivity is expressed in terms of disintegrations per second (dps). The SI unit of radioactivity is Becquerel, abbreviated Bq (1 Bq = 1 dps). The conventional unit of radioactivity is *Curie* (Ci). One Ci is equal to 3.7×10^{10} dps. The typical radioactivity dose administered to patients in Nuclear Medicine investigations is in range of millicurie (mCi) or Mega Becquerel (MBq) [1 mCi = 37 MBq].

In the living tissues, the ionizations caused due to radioactivity result in the deposition of energy, which is quantified in terms of absorbed dose. The SI unit used for absorbed dose is *Gray,* abbreviated Gy (1Gy = 1 Joule/kg). The conventional unit for absorbed dose is rad. One Gy is equivalent to 100 rads (1 Gy = 100 rads). Effective dose is the whole body dose taking into account the type of radiation and sensitivity of organs/tissues. The SI unit of effective dose is Sievert (Sv) and conventional unit is roentgen equivalent man (rem). One Sv is equal to 100 rem. Typical effective dose in Nuclear Medicine and radiological investigations is in range of milli Sieverts (mSv).

The radionuclides are tagged with a specific biologically active molecule or pharmaceutical to form a compound called as *radiopharmaceutical.* The radionuclide helps in external detection/therapeutic effect, while the pharmaceutical component acts as a carrier and determines localization and biodistribution. The term *radiotracer* is also used for radiopharmaceutical as they are administered in micro/nano-molar amounts to "trace" a particular physiological or pathologic process in the body.

The radionuclides emitting gamma rays (high energy photons) are used for imaging, and those undergoing alpha and beta negative decay (particles) are used for therapeutic purposes. Radionuclides emitting positrons (positive electrons, β^+) are used for positron emission tomography (PET). These radionuclides are produced in nuclear reactors, cyclotron or radionuclide generator systems. Tables 1 and 2 show commonly used radionuclides in Nuclear Medicine.

Table 1: Most commonly used diagnostic radionuclides in Nuclear Medicine

Radionuclide	Abbreviation	Decay mode / Energy(MeV)	Half-life
Technetium-99m	^{99m}Tc	γ (0.14)	6 hours
Fluorine-18	^{18}F	β^+ (0.64), EC	110 min.
Gallium-68	^{68}Ga	β^+ (1.9), EC	68 min.
Nitrogen-13	^{13}N	β^+ (1.2), EC	10 min.

γ,Gamma; β^+,Positron; EC,Electron capture; min.,minute.

Table 2: Most commonly used therapeutic radionuclides in Nuclear Medicine

Radionuclide	Abbreviation	Decay mode/Energy (MeV)	Half-life
Iodine-131	^{131}I	β^- (0.606), γ (0.364)	8 days
Lutetium-177	^{177}Lu	β^- (0.497), γ (0.176)	6.7 days
Yttrium-90	^{90}Y	β^- (2.28)	64.1 hours
Rhenium-188	^{188}Re	β^- (2.12), γ (0.155)	16.9 hours
Actinium-225	^{225}Ac	α (5.9)	10 days

β^-, Beta; γ, Gamma; α, alpha.

1.3 Radiation Protection

Due to the ionizing nature of radioactivity, radiation protection principles and regulations have been formulated by the International Commission on Radiological Protection (ICRP) to prevent harm from the use of radiation.

Radiation protection is based on three fundamental principles of justification, optimization and dose limitation. The first principle is that the radiation exposure to an individual should be justified, i.e. the benefits should outweigh the risks associated. Optimisation of radiation exposure, the second principle, is ensured by adopting the concept of 'as low as reasonably achievable' (ALARA). This concept aims at minimising radiation exposure so that maximum benefits are derived with minimum risk. The third principle is the application of dose limits to ensure that no individual is exposed to radiation risk that is too high to be acceptable. There are no radiation exposure limits for patients. However, the principle of justification and optimisation applies to patients to keep their exposure minimum. Effective radiation dose to the patient from most diagnostic nuclear medicine procedures is comparable to radiation dose from radiological investigations using ionising radiation, like computed tomography (*see Appendix*). Good hydration before and after the procedures helps to reduce the overall radiation dose to the patients.

In addition, the radiation exposure to pediatric patients is limited by reducing the administered radioactivity. The radioactivity

(A) to be administered to pediatric patients is calculated using Webster's formula:

$$A = \frac{Age\ of\ patient\ (years) + 1}{Age\ of\ patient\ (years) + 7}\ \text{Adult dose}$$

From the point of view of radiation protection, the main contraindication for nuclear medicine procedures is pregnancy; to avoid radiation exposure to the foetus. Lactation is not a contraindication; however, breastfeeding may need to be temporarily stopped depending upon the radiopharmaceutical administered. In rare circumstances when radioiodine therapy is administered during lactation, complete cessation of lactation is advised.

The external radiation exposure to the occupational workers can be reduced by taking into account three factors: time (T), distance (D) and shielding (S). Spending less time in the vicinity of the radiation source reduces the radiation exposure proportionally. Increasing the distance from the radiation source reduces the exposure by a factor of square of distance. The third essential element is shielding the radioactive source with a material having high atomic number like lead, tungsten or concrete to absorb the radiation. A combination of these factors (TDS) can effectively reduce radiation exposure to safe levels.

1.4 Instrumentation

Dose Calibrator

The radionuclide dose calibrator is used to measure the radiopharmaceutical doses (radioactivity) before patient administration. Dose calibrator is also used for measuring the radioactivity obtained from radionuclide generators, cyclotron, and packages containing radioactive materials and radiopharmaceutical preparations. It is a gas-filled cylinder with a well in the center into which the radioactive sample containing vial or syringe is placed. When gamma rays or other radioactive emissions ionize the gas between the electrodes, ionization current is created, which is used to estimate the amount of radioactivity present in a sample [typically in millicurie (mCi) or Mega Becquerel (MBq) range].

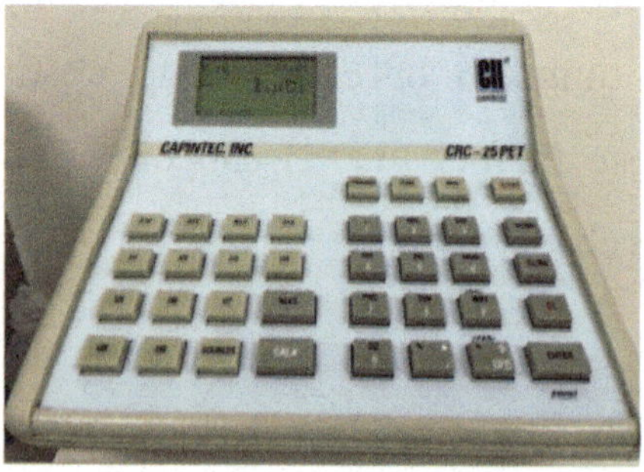

Dose Calibrator

Gamma Camera: Gamma camera, also known as scintillation or Anger camera, is the most commonly used imaging system in nuclear medicine. The gamma camera works on the principle of scintillation, i.e., conversion of the gamma rays that hit the detector (sodium iodide crystals) into light photons, which are amplified and converted into a signal to form an image. Hence, the term 'scintigraphy' is used to refer to most nuclear medicine investigations. The procedure involves the administration of a radiopharmaceutical specific to the organ of interest to the patient. Once the radiopharmaceutical gets trapped/metabolized in the target organ or tissue, the emitted rays are detected using the gamma camera to produce functional images of different organs, like the brain, lungs, thyroid, liver, skeleton, kidneys, etc.

Furthermore, 3-dimensional datasets can be acquired by rotating the detectors around the patient and reconstructed into orthogonal tomographic images. This tomography technique is called Single Photon Emission Computed Tomography (SPECT). Hybrid SPECT-CT systems acquire and fuse SPECT images with CT for better anatomical localisation and characterisation.

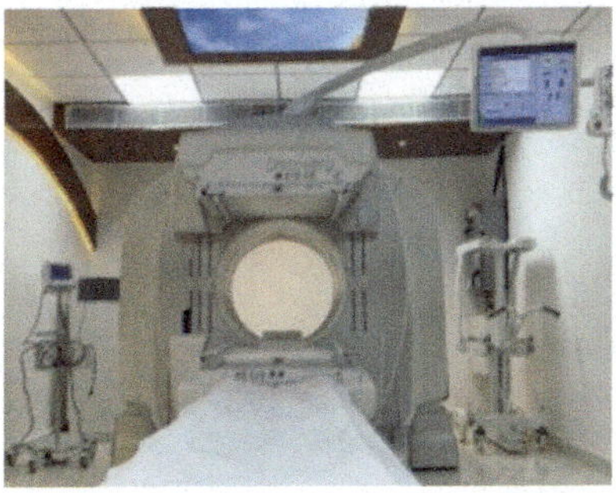

Dual head gamma camera with SPECT-CT

Positron Emission Tomography (PET)

Positron Emission Tomography (PET) is one of the most commonly used imaging technique in Nuclear Medicine, apart from gamma camera. The radiotracers used in PET imaging are positron-emitting radionuclides with a short half-life (e.g., ^{18}F, ^{68}Ga, ^{13}N). After administration of the radiotracer to the patient, positrons are emitted after radioactive decay, and two high-energy gamma rays are created by annihilation, which are simultaneously detected by the PET system. The most commonly used PET radiopharmaceutical is 2-fluoro-2-deoxy-d-glucose (FDG), a glucose analogue with applications in oncological and non-oncological pathologies. Hybrid PET-CT and PET-MR systems provide both functional and anatomical information.

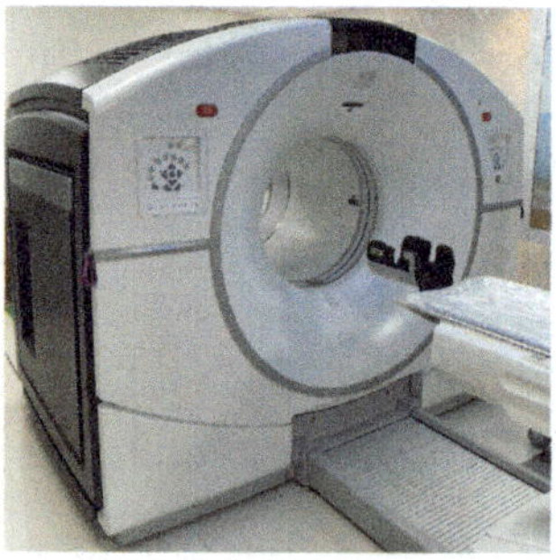

PET-CT scanner

1.5 The Nuclear Medicine Image

One needs to be familiar with the basic characteristics of Nuclear Medicine images to interpret them. Each radiopharmaceutical localizes to different organs of the body and lesions, depending on its mechanism of uptake. The radiotracer emits gamma rays, which are imaged using gamma or PET camera. The physiological distribution of radiotracer seen in the images tells the reader about the radiopharmaceutical used. Broadly, images in Nuclear Medicine are of two types:

1. Planar images
2. Tomographic images

Planar images

These are two-dimensional images, analogous to x-ray films, which show the radiotracer distribution in the organs of interest. For good image resolution, the gamma camera detector needs to be as close to the organ of interest as possible. Therefore, for anteriorly located organs like thyroid, anterior projections (views) are acquired. Similarly, posterior views are acquired for posteriorly located organs, like kidneys. Oblique images can also be acquired. In whole body imaging, both anterior and posterior whole body images are acquired simultaneously using dual detector gamma camera, for example, for skeletal scintigraphy, ^{131}I whole body scan, etc.

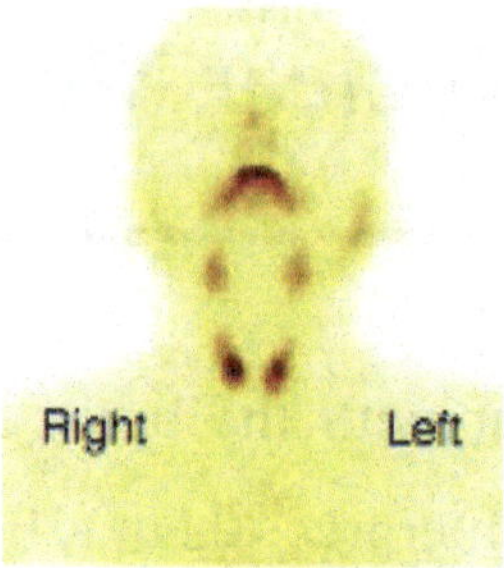

Planar image: Normal ^{99m}Tc-pertechnetate thyroid scan (Static anterior view of the neck)

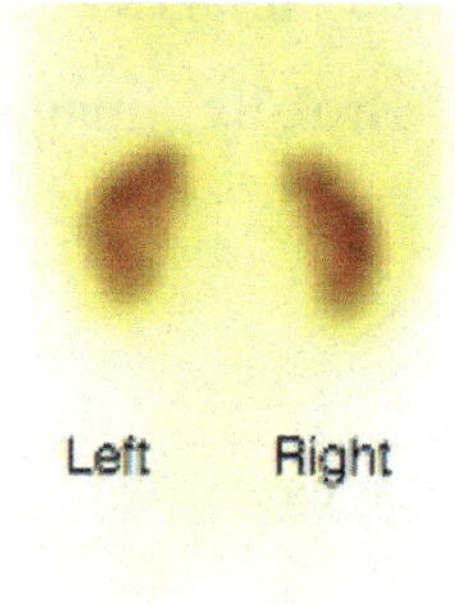

Planar image: Renal scan (Static posterior view of kidneys)

Planar images showing radiotracer distribution in an organ at a particular time are referred to as *static images.* Multiple planar images can be acquired over time after radiotracer injection to generate a sequence of *dynamic images,* which are reviewed to see radiotracer dynamics over-time, for example, excretion of bile or urine. They can be viewed as cinematic (cine) video display. Region of interest (ROI) can be drawn on dynamic images to generate time-activity curves (TACs) showing transit of a tracer in an organ of interest. Images can be seen in different colour scales and window (intensity) levels.

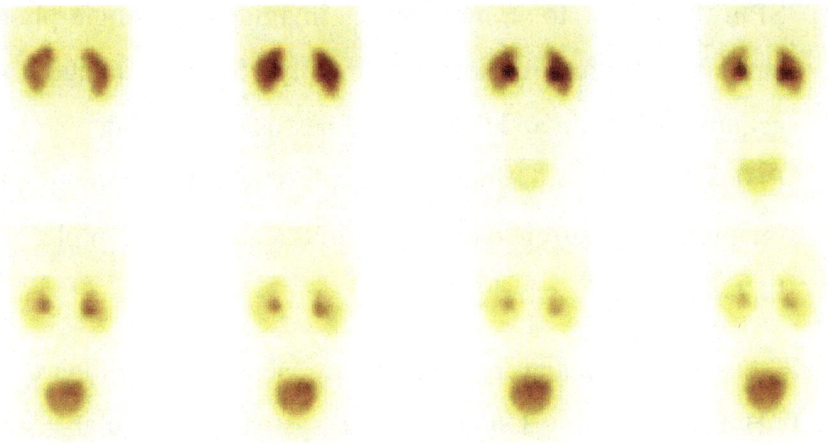

Dynamic planar images: Renal dynamic scan
(Posterior view of the kidneys)

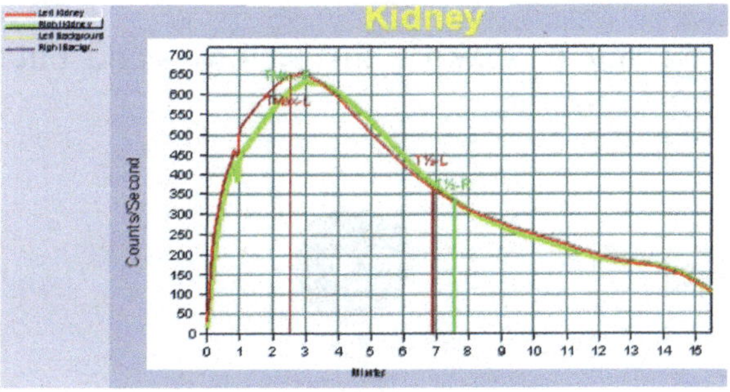

Normal time-activity curves of both kidneys in a renal dynamic scan indicating initial tracer uptake in both kidneys (upslope) followed by clearance of tracer (downslope), indicating non-obstructive urinary clearance.

Tomographic images

Three-dimensional tomographic data is acquired, analogous to CT, and orthogonal images (axial, sagittal, coronal) can be generated. In general, tomographic images provide better image contrast and sensitivity compared to planar images. The two tomographic techniques in Nuclear Medicine are:

1. SPECT refers to tomographic imaging of single-photon gamma emitting radiotracers. Only SPECT images are acquired for brain and myocardial perfusion imaging.
2. PET (Positron emission tomography) refers to tomographic imaging of positron emitting radiotracers, for example, ^{18}F-FDG PET.

PET has better spatial resolution and sensitivity compared to SPECT. Hybrid SPECT-CT and PET-CT systems are available now, which provide both functional and anatomical information. *Maximum intensity projection* (MIP) image refers to 2-dimensional representation of volumetric 3-dimensional data to represent voxels with the highest value in all directions. The MIP image give a quick whole body assessment, making the lesions stand out and easier to detect.

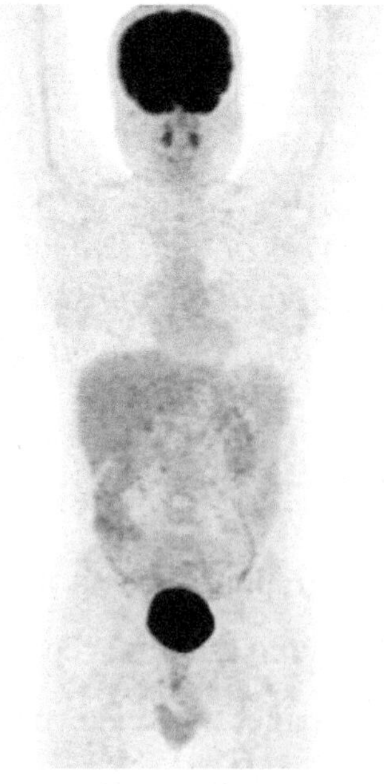

^{18}F-FDG PET MIP image
(Note the normal physiological tracer distribution)

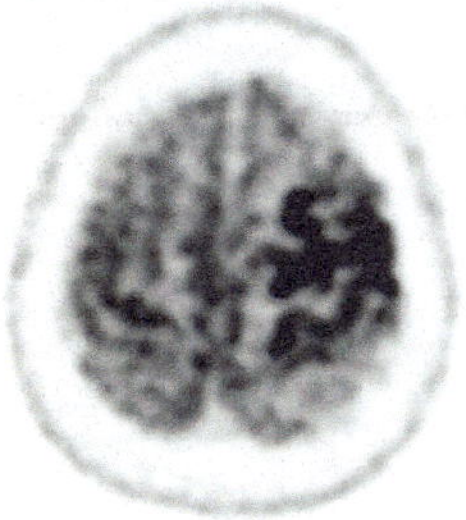

Transaxial ^{18}F-FDG PET image of the brain (with lesion)

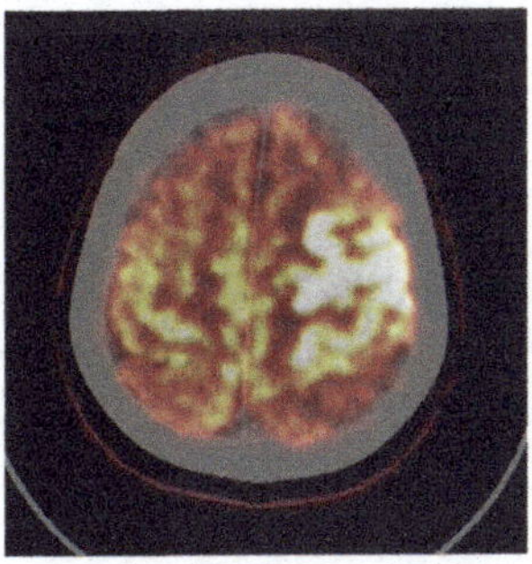

Transaxial ^{18}F-FDG fused PET-CT image of the brain (with lesion)

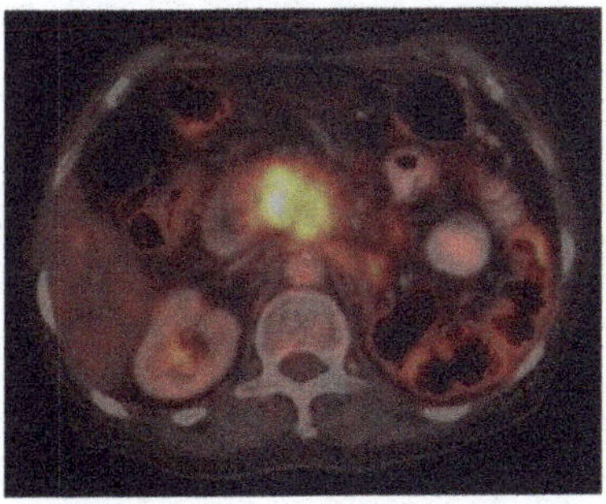

Transaxial ^{18}F-FDG fused PET-CT image (Pancreatic cancer)

Section 2

Endocrinology

Dr. Venkata Subramanian K

Prof. Anish Bhattacharya

2.1 Radioactive Iodine Uptake (RAIU)

Mechanism:

- Radioactive iodine (RAI) is taken up by the sodium-iodide symporter (NIS) in the thyroid gland and organified. RAI uptake study (RAIU) is used for quantification of the radioiodine uptake within the thyroid gland. The uptake is quantified using a thyroid uptake probe with serial measurements at 2 and 24 hours.
- The advantage of performing RAIU over ^{99m}Tc-pertechnetate thyroid scan is that RAI is both trapped and organified in the thyroid gland, while pertechnetate is only trapped.

Patient preparation: Fasting for 4 hours. Discontinue thyroxine, anti thyroid drugs and iodine-containing medications/ointments/ supplements. No intravenous iodinated contrast study in the last 6-8 weeks.

Radiopharmaceutical	^{131}I–Sodium Iodide	^{123}I–Sodium Iodide
Administration route	Oral	Oral
Activity (Dose for adults)	5-10μCi (0.18-0.37 MBq)	50-100 μCi (1.8-3.7 MBq)
Imaging	Not possible	Possible

μCi, microcurie; MBq, Mega Becquerel.

Indications:

- To differentiate causes of thyrotoxicosis – Hyper-functioning thyroid gland (Graves' disease, toxic adenoma, toxic MNG) vs. destruction of gland (thyroiditis)/.
- Estimate dose of ^{131}I RAI therapy for treatment of hyperthyroidism (*section 11.1*).
- Diagnosis of organification defect as the cause of hypothyroidism in children (Dyshormonogenesis).

Patterns of RAIU values	
Normal RAIU	Vary with the level of iodine sufficiency in the population. In iodine sufficient population, 2 hour RAIU ranges between 1–6% and 24 hour RAIU between 6-18%.
High RAIU (Progressively increasing 2 and 24 hours values)	Seen in Graves' disease, toxic MNG, toxic adenoma, thyroid stimulating hormone (TSH)/ human chorionic gonadotropin secreting tumours.
High RAIU (High 2 hour value with normal or low 24 hours value)	Seen in Graves' disease with gland showing rapid iodide turnover.
Low RAIU	Seen in thyrotoxic phase of thyroiditis, exogenous thyroxine stimulation and struma ovarii.

Perchlorate Discharge Test

- Iodine trapped by the thyroid gland undergoes enzymatic organification. After binding to tyrosine residues in thyroglobulin, iodine cannot washout from the thyroid gland.
- Defective enzymes or thyroglobulin lead to organification defect and thyroid dysfunction.
- RAI trapped in thyroid remains in inorganic form and exits the thyroid gland following administration of perchlorate (which is demonstrated as decrease in the RAIU).
- RAIU is estimated at baseline and two hours after perchlorate administration (400mg orally in adults).

Interpretation

- No organification defect - <10% drop in RAIU from baseline.
- Partial organification defect - 10-90% drop in RAIU.
- Total organification defect - >90% drop in RAIU.

2.2 Thyroid Scintigraphy

Mechanism: Radiopharmaceutical concentrates in functioning thyroid tissue (trapped) with the amount of tracer concentration proportional to NIS expression. NIS expression depends on the stimulation of the thyroid gland by TSH or other similar hormones/antibodies that mimic TSH. RAI is organified while pertechnetate is not.

Patient preparation: Discontinue thyroxine, anti thyroid drugs, iodine-containing medications/ointments/supplements, and no iodinated contrast study 6-8 weeks prior to the scan. 4 hour fasting before ^{123}I-sodium iodide scan.

Radiopharmaceutical	^{99m}Tc–Pertechnetate	^{123}I–Sodium Iodide
Administration route	Intravenous	Oral
Activity (Dose for adults)	4-5 mCi(148-185 MBq)	200-400 µCi(7.4-14.8 MBq)

mCi, Millicurie;µCi, microcurie; MBq, Mega Becquerel.

Indications:

- In children/adults:
    - To look for the cause of thyrotoxicosis – Hyperfunctioning gland (Graves' disease, toxic adenoma, toxic MNG) vs. destruction of the gland (thyroiditis)/exogenous thyroid stimulation.

- Evaluation and characterization of thyroid nodules identified clinically or on radiological imaging.
  - Characterization into hot, warm or cold nodule.
- Whole body scan in thyroid cancer.

- In children:
  - In hypothyroid children – to look for the cause (thyroid dysgenesis vs. dyshormonogenesis).
  - To look for ectopic thyroid tissue (lingual thyroid, midline neck swelling, etc.).

Common imaging patterns	
Normal ^{99m}Tc-pertechnetate thyroid scan *Both lobes of the thyroid are symmetrical in size and shape, showing homogeneous tracer activity. Salivary glands and background tracer activity are well visualized. ^{99m}Tc-pertechnetate uptake can also be quantified (Normal 0.5-4%)*	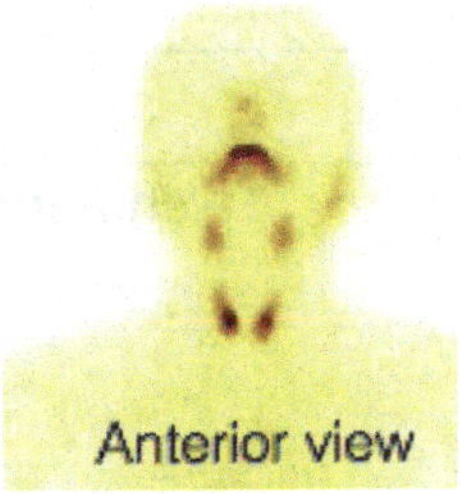
Graves' disease (Increased NIS expression due to TSH receptor stimulating antibodies) • *Both lobes of the thyroid gland are enlarged with diffuse increased tracer activity.* • *Background and salivary gland activity are suppressed.*	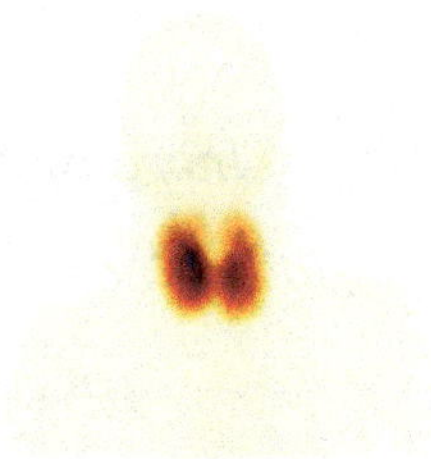

<table>
<tr><td colspan="2">Subacute thyroiditis and exogenous thyroid stimulation (secondary to gland destruction/ suppressed TSH levels)
<ul><li>Negligible tracer activity in the region of the thyroid gland.</li><li>Background tracer activity is increased.</li></ul></td><td>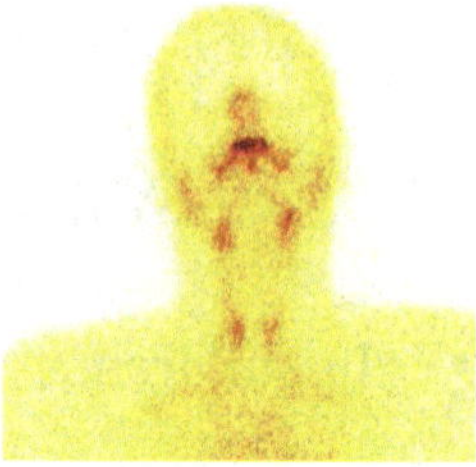</td></tr>
<tr><td>Cold nodule
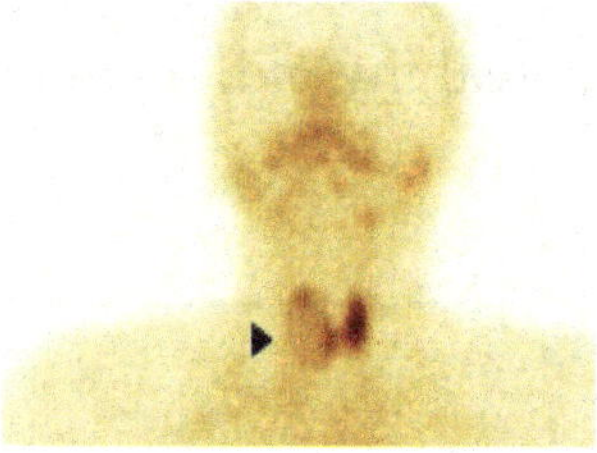
15-20% malignant</td><td>Hot nodule (Toxic adenoma)
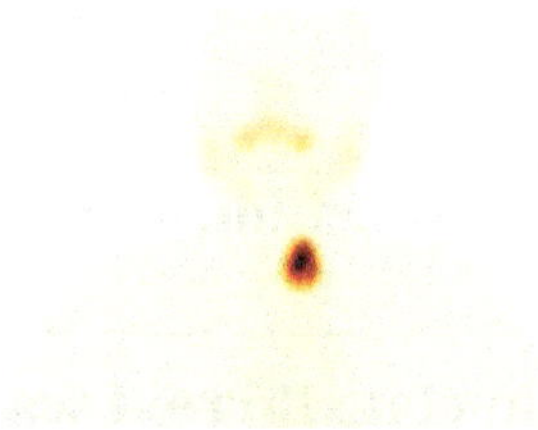
<1% malignant</td><td>Toxic MNG
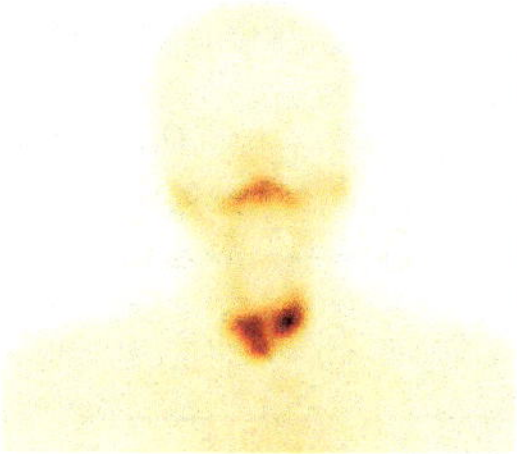</td></tr>
<tr><td colspan="3">Hypothyroid children</td></tr>
<tr><td colspan="2">Dyshormonogenesis
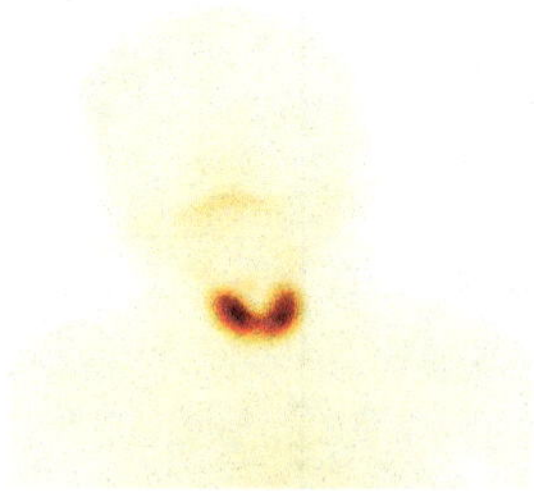
Increased trapping of iodine/pertechnetate but not organified.</td><td>Thyroid agenesis
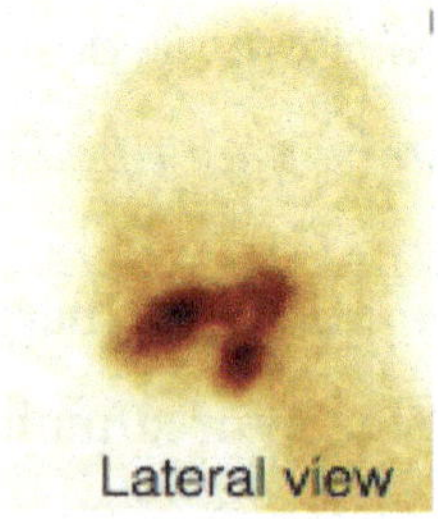

Absent tracer activity in the thyroid bed with increased background activity.</td></tr>
</table>

2.3 Parathyroid Scintigraphy

Mechanism:

Dual-phase ^{99m}Tc-sestamibi parathyroid scintigraphy

- ^{99m}Tc-sestamibi is a lipophilic cation, taken up and retained in the abundant mitochondria-containing cells in the parathyroid adenoma (mostly oxyphil cells). Normal parathyroid glands are not visualized.

- ^{99m}Tc-sestamibi concentrates in normal thyroid tissue, normal parathyroid tissue, and parathyroid adenomas in the early phase (~10 minutes post-injection) while parathyroid adenomas retain the tracer till the delayed phase imaging (after 1-2 hours). SPECT/CT helps in better anatomical localization.

- To subtract thyroid gland activity, dual tracer subtraction imaging with ^{99m}Tc-sestamibi and ^{99m}Tc-pertechnetate can also be done.

^{18}F – Fluorocholine PET:

- Localizes parathyroid adenomas by targeting the increased choline metabolism in tumours. Choline is used for cell membrane phosphatidylcholine synthesis.
- Useful when ^{99m}Tc-sestamibi scan is negative or equivocal.

Patient preparation:

No special preparation needed.

Radiopharmaceutical	^{99m}Tc–Sestamibi	^{18}F-Fluorocholine
Administration route	Intravenous	Intravenous
Dose (for adults)	20 mCi (740 MBq)	5 mCi (185 MBq)

mCi, Millicurie; MBq, Mega Becquerel.

Indication: For localization of parathyroid adenoma.

Common Imaging patterns		
^{99m}Tc–Sestamibi dual-phase parathyroid scintigraphy		
Normal scan *Thyroid and salivary gland activity is seen in the early phase. Thyroid gland activity washes out in the delayed phase. No focal tracer retention is noted.*	**Early phase (at 15 min)** 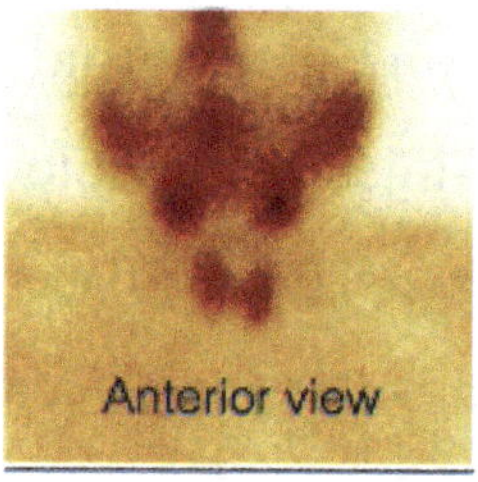	**Delayed phase (at 2 hours)** 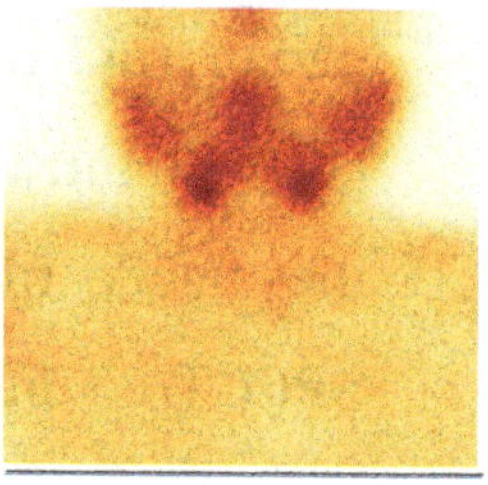
Parathyroid adenoma		
Early phase 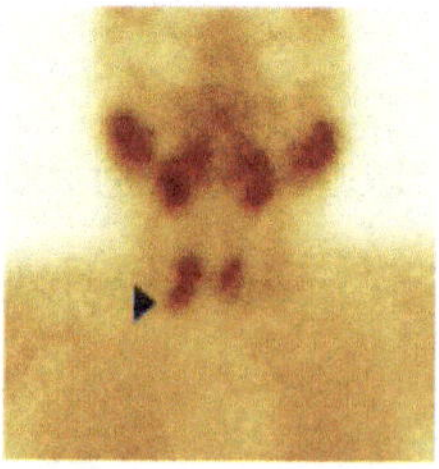 *Focus increased tracer activity on early image (at lower pole of right lobe of thyroid).*	**Delayed phase** 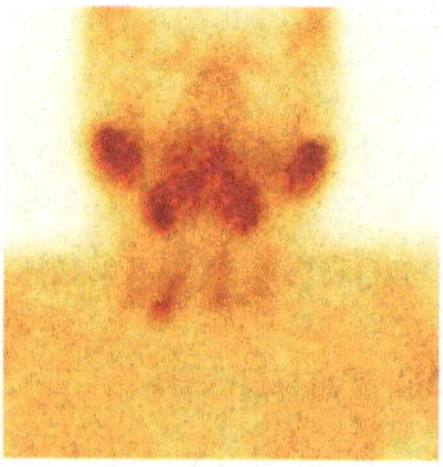 *Slower washout in the delayed phase, in contrast to thyroid uptake.*	**SPECT/CT** 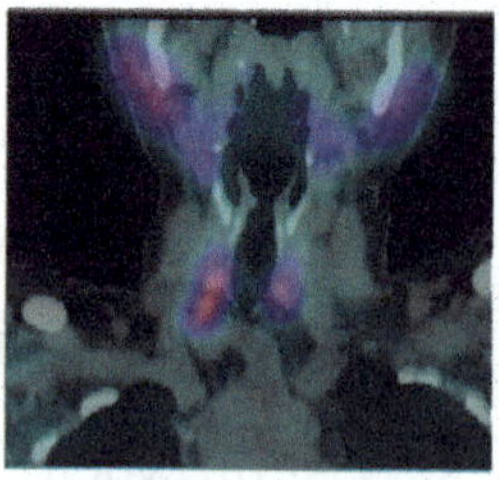 *Better anatomical localization.*

^{18}F- Fluorocholine PET-CT		
• **Normal scan** • *No tracer activity in the thyroid gland with physiological tracer uptake in salivary glands.* • *Focal increased tracer uptake is seen in* parathyroid adenoma.	**Normal scan** 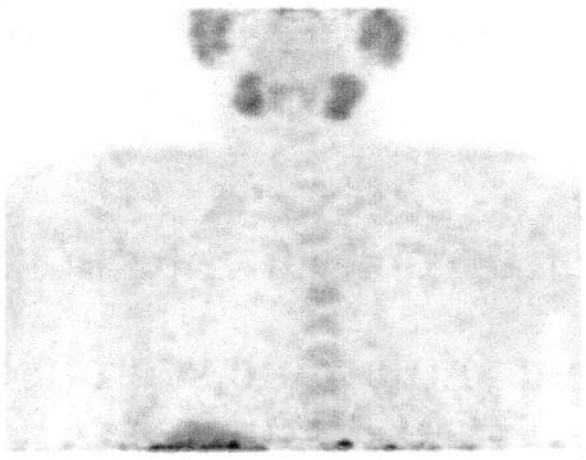	**Parathyroid adenoma** 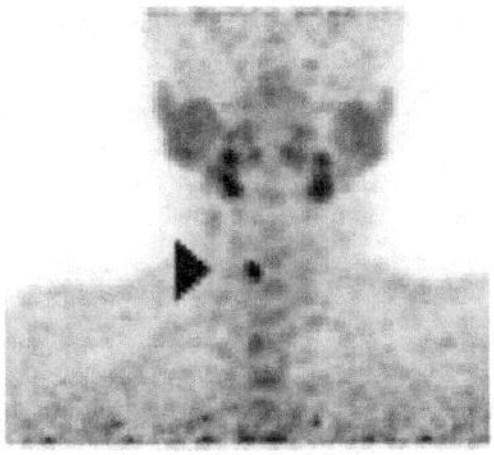

2.4 MIBG Scintigraphy

Mechanism:

- MIBG stands for metaiodobenzylguanidine, which is an analogue of noradrenaline and guanethidine. MIBG is labeled with ^{131}I or ^{123}I.
- Tracer localization is dependent upon the adrenergic innervation and the level of catecholamine secretion in tumors.

Patient preparation:

- Drugs interfering with the adrenergic system should be stopped (selected anti-hypertensives, anti-psychotics, tricyclic anti-depressants, opioids, tramadol and sympathomimetic drugs).
- Stable oral iodine is administered to block the thyroid gland and prevent the accumulation of free radioiodine.

Radiopharmaceutical	^{131}I-MIBG	^{123}I-MIBG
Administration	Intravenous	Intravenous
Activity (Dose for adults)	1 mCi (37 MBq)	10 mCi (370 MBq)

mCi, Millicurie; MBq, Mega Becquerel.

Indications:

- For detection and staging of pheochromocytoma, paraganglioma, carcinoid, neuroblastoma and medullary thyroid cancer.

- For planning and assessing response to ^{131}I-MIBG radionuclide therapy (*see Section 11.9*).

- To assess sympathetic innervation of the myocardium in heart failure and Parkinson's disease.

<table>
<tr><th colspan="4">Common imaging patterns</th></tr>
<tr><td colspan="4">
<ul>
<li>Whole-body images are acquired, which show normal physiological uptake of ^{131}I-MIBG in the liver, salivary glands, myocardium, and excretion into the urinary bladder.</li>
<li>Abnormal lesions are seen as focal areas of increased tracer uptake.</li>
<li>SPECT/CT can be done for anatomical localization.</li>
</ul>
</td></tr>
<tr><th colspan="2">Normal ^{131}I-MIBG Scan</th><th colspan="2">Right adrenal pheochromocytoma</th></tr>
<tr><td>Anterior</td><td>Posterior</td><td>Anterior</td><td>Posterior</td></tr>
<tr><td>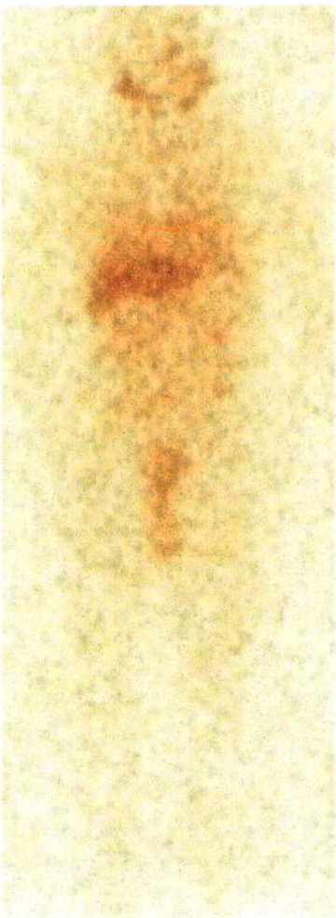</td><td>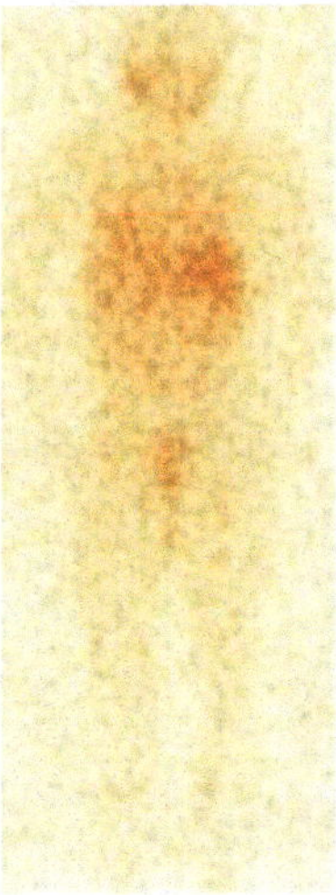</td><td>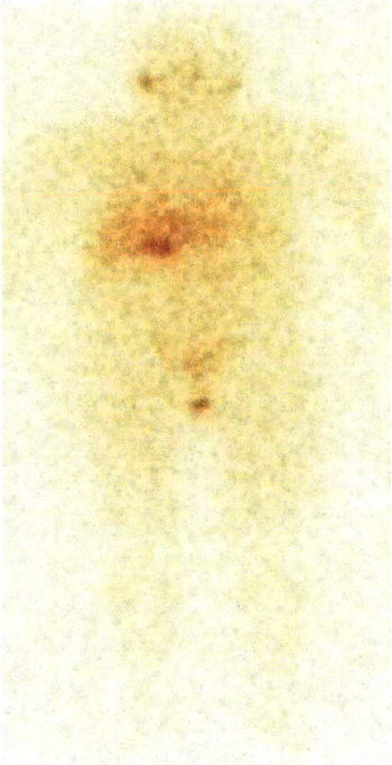</td><td>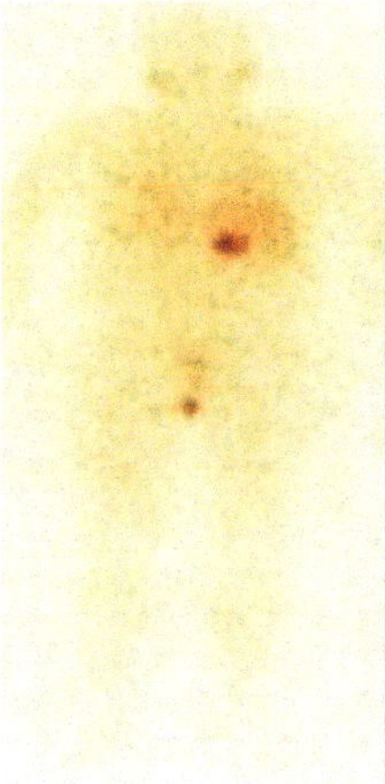</td></tr>
</table>

Section 3

Skeletal Scintigraphy and ^{18}F-Fluoride PET

Dr. Yamini Mathur
Prof. Anish Bhattacharya

3 Skeletal Scintigraphy & ^{18}F-Fluoride PET

Mechanism:

- Radiopharmaceutical uptake occurs by chemisorption on the hydroxyapatite mineral component of the osseous bone matrix.
- The tracer uptake is increased at sites of increased osteoblastic activity, e.g. sclerotic metastasis and osteomyelitis. On the other hand, the tracer uptake is reduced at sites of osteolytic lesions, bone cysts, etc.

Patient preparation:

- No special preparation is needed. Ensure good hydration.

Radiopharmaceutical	**^{99m}Tc - Methylene Diphosphonate (MDP)**	**^{18}F-Sodium Fluoride (NaF) PET**
Administration	Intravenous	Intravenous
Dose for adults	20 mCi (740 MBq)	5-10 mCi (185-370 MBq)
Time of delayed imaging	2-4 hours	0.5-1.5 hours
Image quality	Good	Excellent

mCi, Millicurie; MBq, Mega Becquerel.

Different components of the pathophysiology can be assessed in a three-phase ^{99m}Tc-MDP bone scan:

Phase	Imaging time	Interpretation
Flow phase	Immediately after injection	Relative blood flow
Blood pool phase	1 minute after injection	Blood pool in the soft tissues
Delayed	2-4 hours after injection	Bone turnover

Indications:

- **Malignant diseases**
  - Primary bone tumours or to look for osteoblastic metastasis.
  - Patient selection for metastatic bone pain palliation radionuclide therapy (*see section 11.5*).
- **Benign bone diseases**
  - Osteomyelitis (acute/chronic)
  - Trauma- Fracture, stress fracture, stress reaction, etc.
  - Prosthesis evaluation (Infection vs. aseptic loosening)
  - Metabolic bone disease
  - Bone dysplasias
  - Avascular necrosis
  - Patient selection for radiosynovectomy (see *section 11.7*)

SPECT-CT is helpful for evaluation of lesions in complex anatomical sites like vertebra, skull and pelvic bones.

Common Imaging Patterns

Normal ^{99m}Tc–MDP bone scan

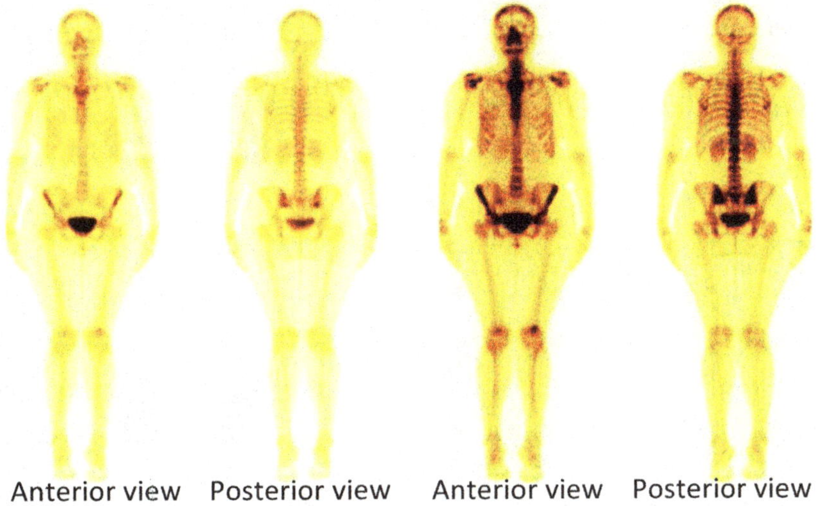

Whole-body images showing physiological tracer uptake in the skeleton. Excretion via kidneys into urinary bladder is seen.

Multiple skeletal metastasis on ^{99m}Tc–MDP bone scan

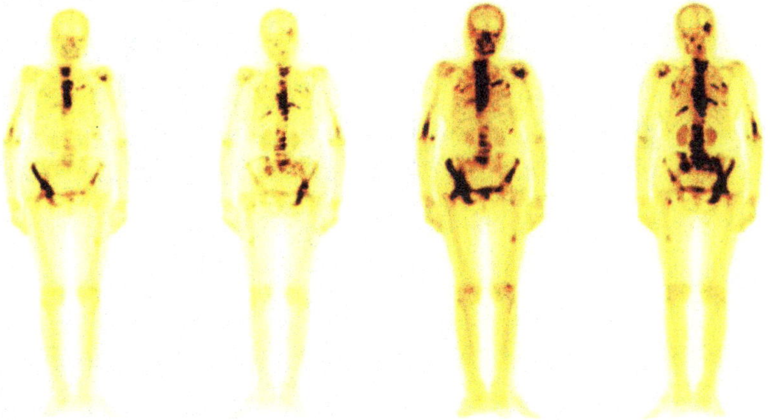

Whole-body images showing focal areas of increased tracer uptake in multiple skeletal sites, suggestive of skeletal metastasis.

Three-phase ^{99m}Tc–MDP bone scan

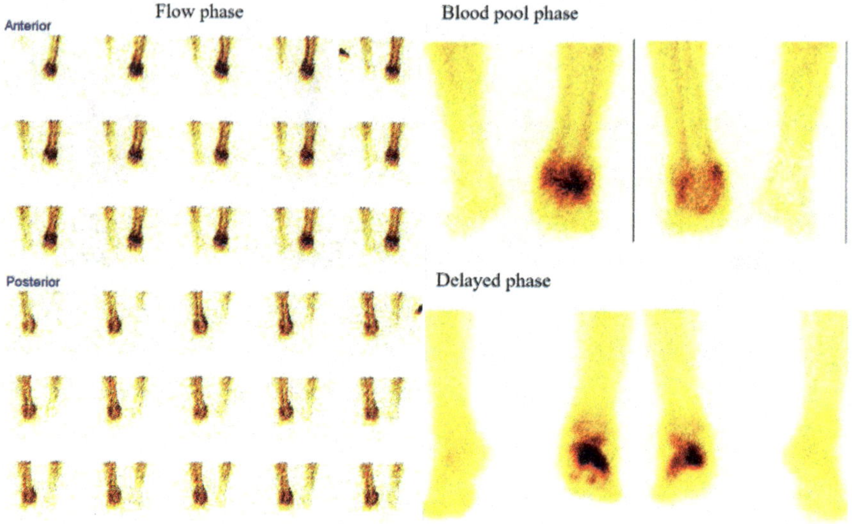

Bilateral lower legs and feet images showing increased perfusion, soft tissue pooling, and osteoblastic activity in the left foot bones, suggestive of active bony infection/inflammation.

Normal ^{18}F-NaF PET scan

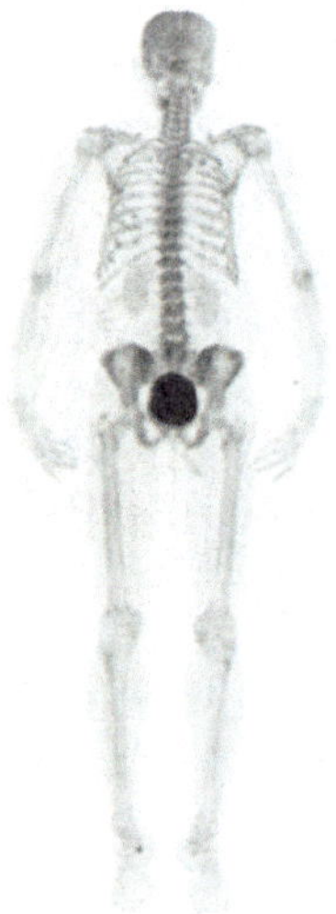

^{18}F-NaF PET MIP image showing physiological tracer distribution in skeleton.

Fibrous Dysplasia

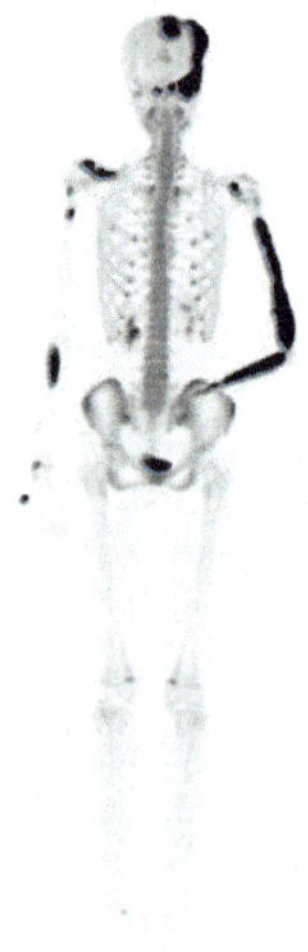

^{18}F-NaF PET MIP image showing increased osteoblastic activity in skull, shoulder and upper limb bones - Polyostotic Fibrous Dysplasia.

Section 4

Urinary System

Dr. Anwin Joseph K
Prof. Anish Bhattacharya

4.1 Dynamic Renal Scintigraphy

Mechanism:

- Radiopharmaceuticals cleared by kidneys either by glomerular filtration or tubular secretion are used to assess renal function and urinary clearance.
- Tubular agents have greater renal extraction than glomerular agents, and have better kidney to background ratio, even at moderate renal impairment, and are the preferred imaging agents.
- Glomerular agents are used for Glomerular Filtration Rate (GFR) estimation.

Radiopharmaceutical	Route of administration	Dose	Mechanism
^{99m}Tc-DTPA (Diethylenetriamine pentaacetate)	Intravenous	1-5 mCi (37-185 MBq)	Glomerular filtration (100%)
^{99m}Tc-MAG3 (mercaptoacetyltriglycine)	Intravenous	1-5 mCi (37-185 MBq)	Tubular secretion (100%)

^{99m}Tc-EC (L, L-ethylene dicysteine)	Intravenous	1-5 mCi (37-185 MBq)	Tubular secretion (83%)

mCi, Millicurie; MBq, Mega Becquerel.

Diuretic Protocols and Dose (for assessing urinary clearance):

Diuretic Protocols	Furosemide can be given 15 min prior to radiotracer (F-15), with the radiotracer (F0) or 10 minutes after radiotracer injection (F+10)
Adult dose	Furosemide 0.5 mg/kg (40 mg usual dose) i.v.
Paediatric dose	Furosemide - 1.0 mg/kg i.v.

Indications:

- **To look for renal obstruction;**
    - In patients with clinical or imaging findings suspicious for obstruction to renal outflow tract.
- **To measure the differential renal function in renal pathologies;**
    - To set a baseline assessment and for follow-up.
    - Aid in surgical decision-making.
- **To estimate the GFR/Effective renal plasma flow (ERPF);**
    - Kidney donors/post-transplant assessment.
    - Pre-bone marrow transplant workup.
    - Radionuclide therapy workup.
    - Nephrotoxicity monitoring.
- **Renal trauma/surgical complications;**

- **Renal transplant evaluation;**
    - Differentiation of Acute tubular necrosis (ATN) vs. Acute Rejection (AR).
    - Obstruction/Leak/characterization of collections.
- **Evaluation of renovascular hypertension.**

Procedure

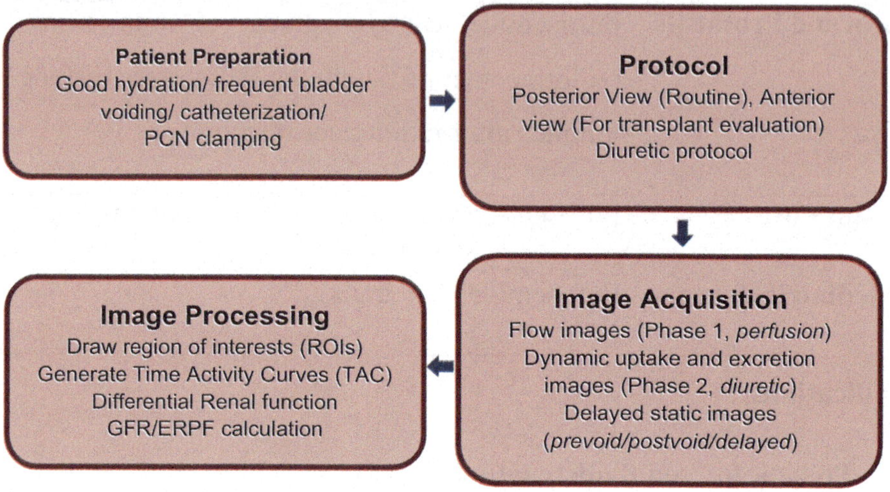

Factors affecting Renogram curve

- Dehydration
- Injection extravasation
- Patient motion
- Increased urinary bladder pressure
- Recent contrast study
- Vesicoureteral reflux during scan

Common Imaging Patterns

Normal ^{99m}Tc-EC Renal Dynamic Scan images

(Posterior view)

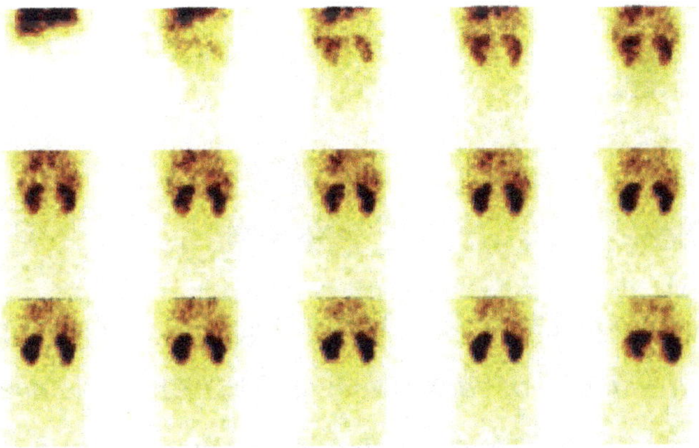

Phase 1 images showing normal blood-flow to both kidneys.

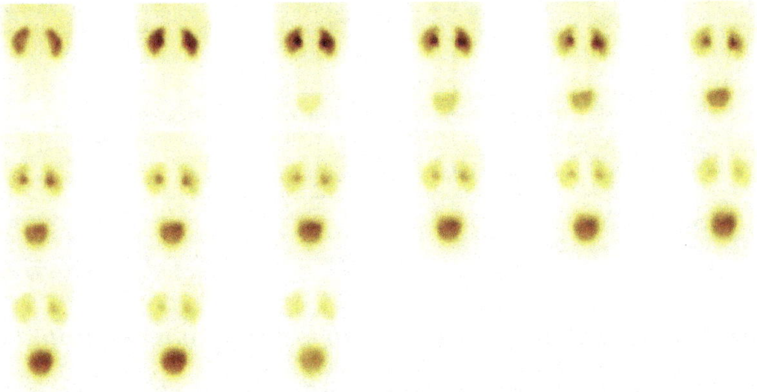

Phase 2 images showing normal cortical uptake (function) and excretion from both kidneys. Note the filling of the urinary bladder over time.

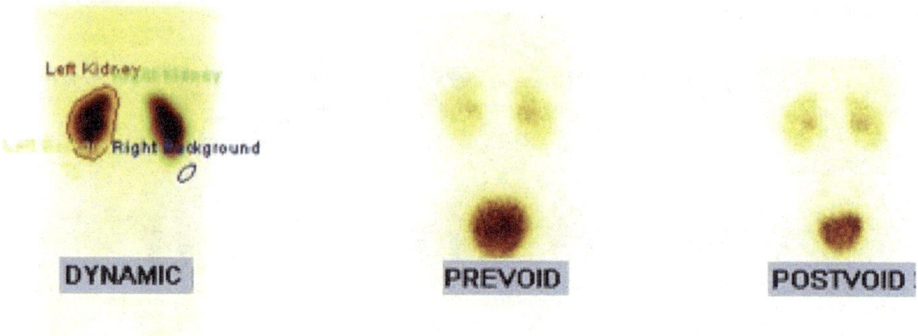

ROIs placed on kidneys in 2-3 min image for processing (Normal differential function of each kidney is 50±5%), Static pre-void and post-void images showing good tracer clearance.

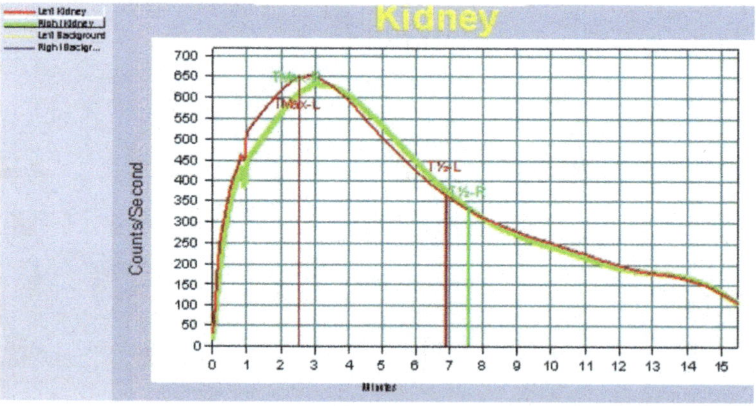

Normal time activity curves of both kidneys showing initial tracer uptake in both kidneys (upslope) followed by clearance of tracer (downslope), indicating non-obstructive urinary clearance. An up-sloping curve without significant tracer clearance suggests urinary tract obstruction.

^{99m}Tc-EC Renal Dynamic Scan showing Pelviureteric junction obstruction (PUJO)

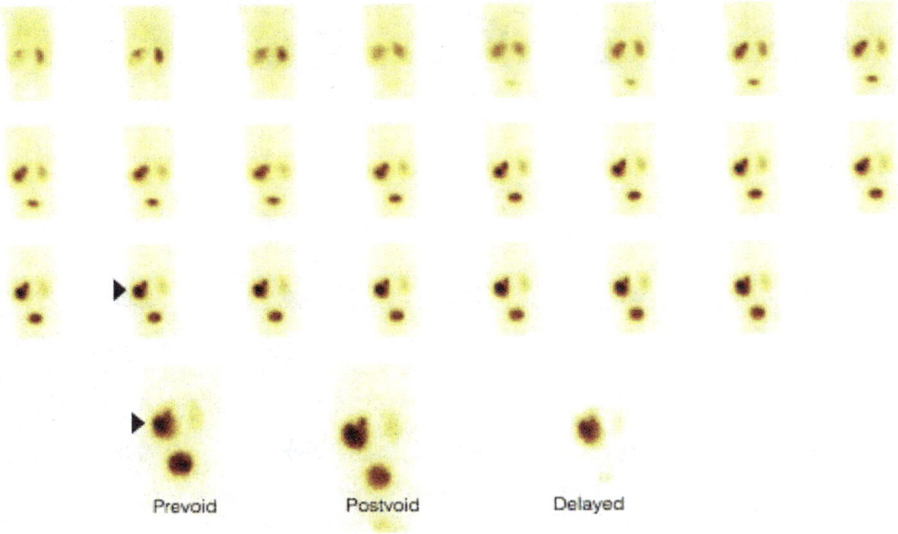

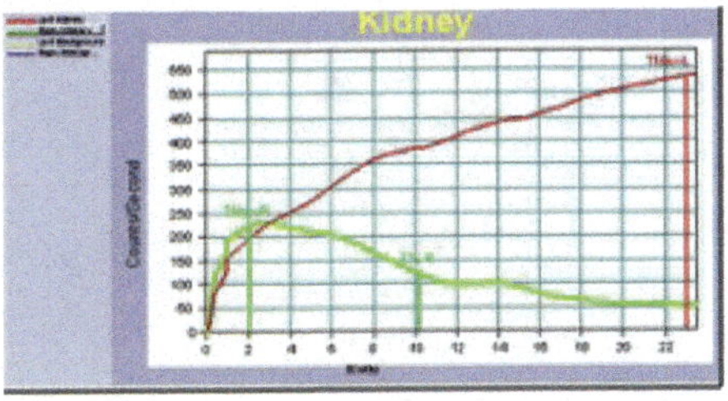

Hydronephrotic left kidney showing impaired perfusion and cortical uptake (denoting impaired function), with dynamic and static images showing significant tracer retention in the dilated left pelvicalyceal system (arrowhead) till 3 hours image and uprising renogram curve (red curve), suggestive of left obstructed drainage (PUJO). Right kidney shows normal function and non-obstructive drainage (green curve).

^{99m}Tc-EC Renal Dynamic Scan (Duplex collecting system with obstruction of one moiety)

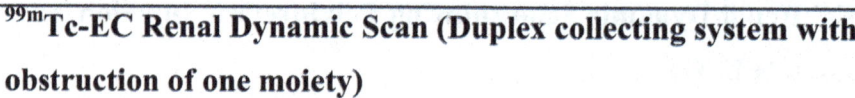

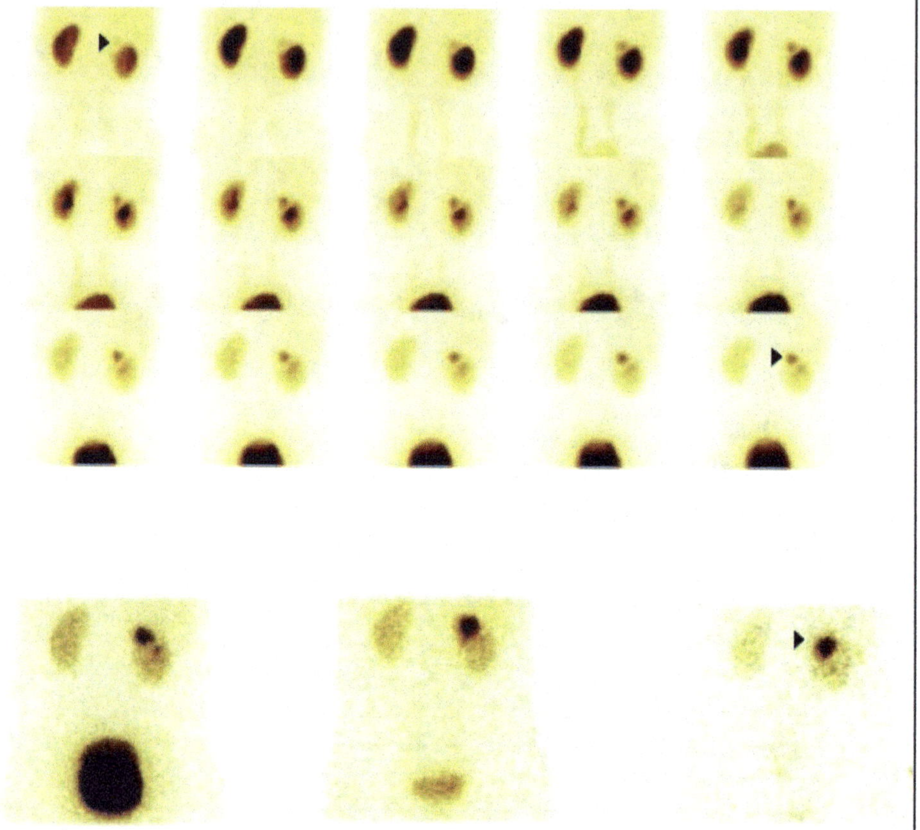

Duplex right kidney with hydronephrotic upper moiety having impaired function and obstructed drainage. Lower moiety and left kidney are showing good cortical uptake and unobstructed drainage.

^{99m}Tc-EC scan of a renal transplant (Anterior view)

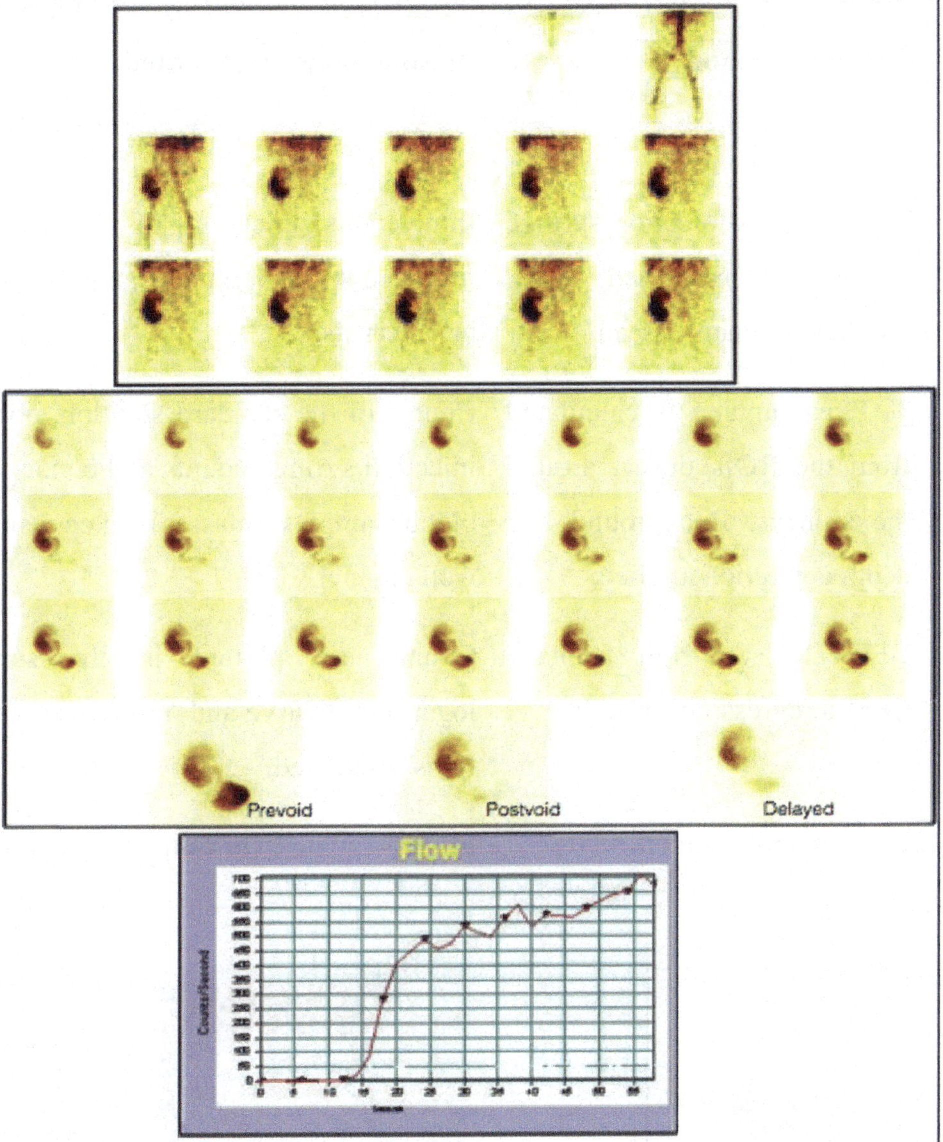

Good perfusion of transplant kidney with significant cortical retention of tracer till 3-hour delayed image - suggestive of ATN.

4.2 Glomerular Filtration Rate (GFR)

Camera Method	Plasma Sampling method
^{99m}Tc-DTPA is used	^{99m}Tc-DTPA or ^{51}Cr-EDTA used.
Pre- and post-injection syringe counts are measured along with renal dynamic scan.	Intravenous injection of the tracer followed by 2-3 blood samples at 1 hr. intervals.
% Renal uptake is calculated from the ROIs drawn around the kidneys. Background and depth correction applied.	Counts of the standard solution, post-injection syringe counts and counts of blood samples (plasma) taken using well counter.
GFR calculated from % uptake using a regression formula.	Counts are plotted in the semi logarithmic curve and Y-intercept and $t_{1/2}$ is calculated.
Usually underestimates GFR.	More accurate than camera method.

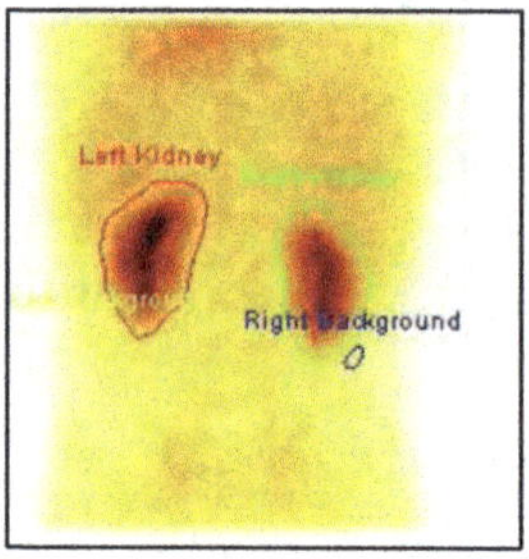

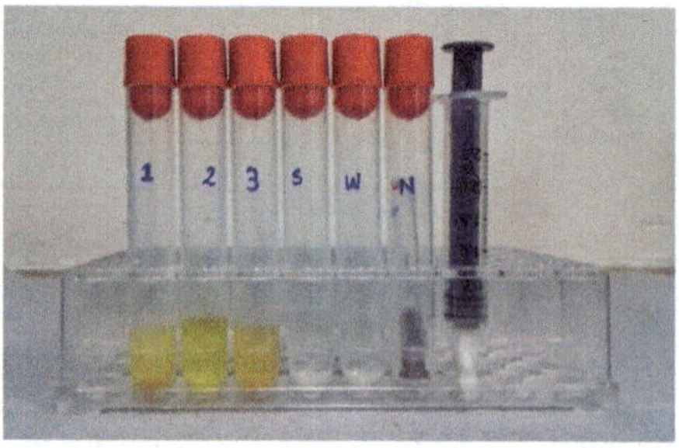

4.3 Radionuclide Cystography

Mechanism: Radionuclide Cystography (RC)

- Radiotracer is filled into the urinary bladder and imaging done during filling, voiding and postvoid phases.

Types:

Indirect RC	Direct RC
Done similar to or as a part of dynamic renal scintigraphy.	Radiotracer with normal saline is used to fill the urinary bladder through catheter/suprapubic injection.
Glomerular/tubular agent given intravenously. Dose is same as diuretic renography.	^{99m}Tc-sulphur colloid is used. Infants 0.25-0.5mCi (9.3-18.5 MBq) Children 0.5-1.0 mCi (18.5-37 MBq)
The bladder gets filled by the tracer through natural route.	Reflux during all the three (filling/voiding/postvoid) phases can be detected.
Upper tract stasis may interfere with the interpretation.	Quantification of post-void residual volume is possible.
Reflux during the filling phase cannot be detected.	Risk of infection is there.

Indications:

- Initial diagnosis of Vesicoureteral reflux (VUR).
- Follow-up of VUR;
    - Assess for spontaneous resolution.
    - Post-medical/surgical management.
- Quantification of post-void residual urine in the bladder.

Grading of reflux:

DRC Reflux Grade	Radiological grade	Reflux level
A	I	Ureter
B	II-III	Pelvis
C	IV-V	Pelvis with dilatation

Common imaging patterns

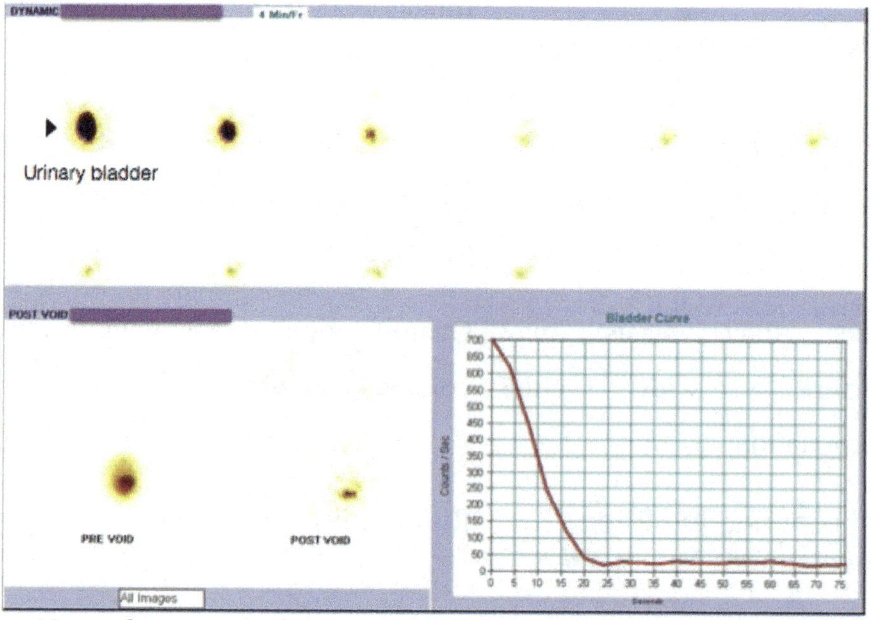

Normal Direct Radionuclide Cystography showing no VUR.

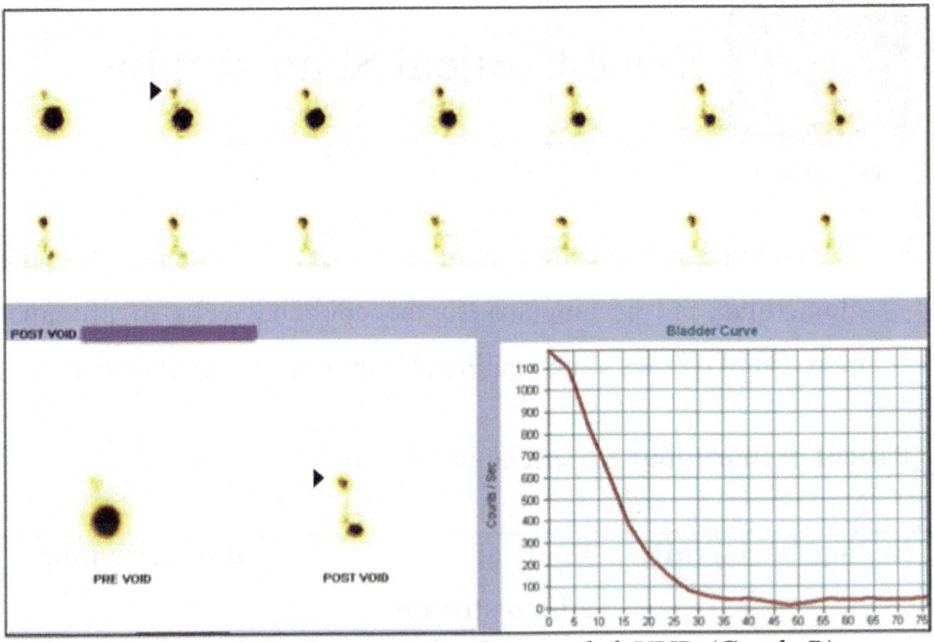

Direct Radionuclide Cystography showing left VUR (Grade B)

4.4 Renal Cortical Scintigraphy

Mechanism:

- ^{99m}Tc-Dimercaptosuccinic acid (DMSA) is filtered by the glomerulus and accumulates in the epithelial cells of proximal convoluted tubules via megalin/cubulin-mediated endocytosis.

Patient preparation: No special preparation is required.

Radiopharmaceutical	Route of administration	Dose for adults
^{99m}Tc DMSA (III)	Intravenous	0.5-3 mCi (18.5-111 MBq)

mCi, Millicurie; MBq, Mega Becquerel.

Indications:

- Evaluation and follow-up of pyelonephritic changes/cortical scars in patients with VUR, recurrent urinary tract infection or lower urinary tract abnormalities.
- Diagnosis and assessment of renal function in congenital renal abnormalities including ectopic kidney, horseshoe kidney, agenesis and multicystic kidney disease.
- Characterization of the renal masses.

Imaging: Planar, pinhole imaging (high resolution) or SPECT/CT.

Common Imaging patterns

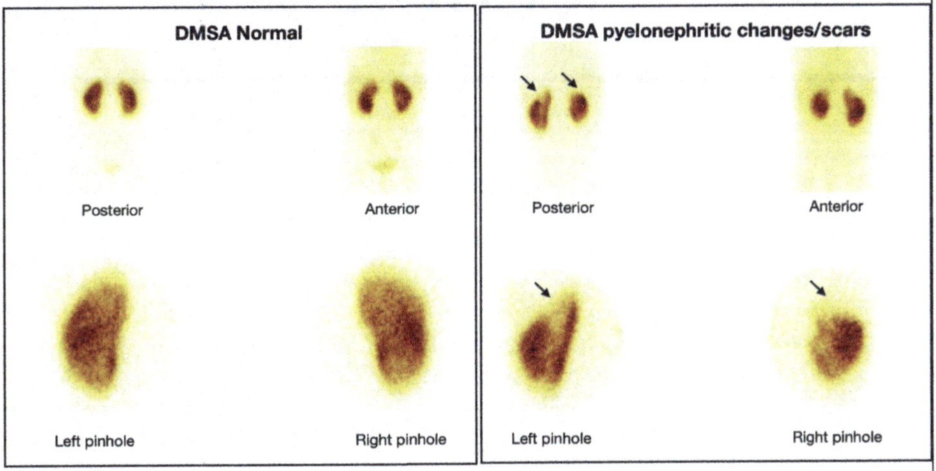
DMSA Normal
Posterior
Anterior
Left pinhole
Right pinhole
DMSA pyelonephritic changes/scars
Posterior
Anterior
Left pinhole
Right pinhole

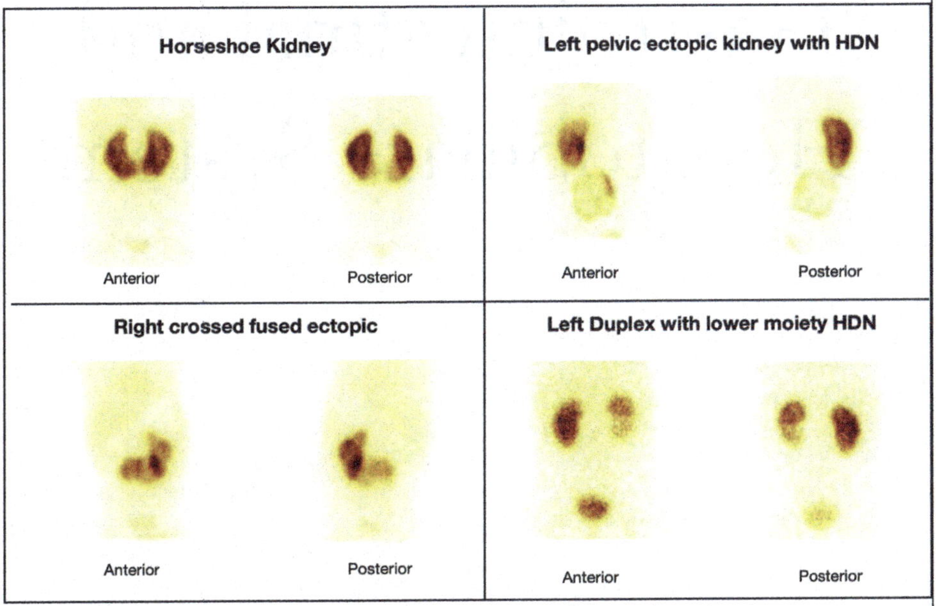
Horseshoe Kidney
Anterior
Posterior
Left pelvic ectopic kidney with HDN
Anterior
Posterior
Right crossed fused ectopic
Anterior
Posterior
Left Duplex with lower moiety HDN
Anterior
Posterior

Section 5

Gastrointestinal and Hepatobiliary System

Dr. Karthikeyan
Dr. Harmandeep Singh
Prof. Anish Bhattacharya

5.1 Gastroesophageal Reflux Scintigraphy

Gastroesophageal reflux disease (GERD) is a medical disorder that mainly presents as heartburn. Other complications like laryngitis can also occur. Gastroesophageal reflux scintigraphy (also known as *milk scan*) is a non-invasive imaging procedure that aids in the diagnosis and quantification of GERD.

Mechanism: The radiopharmaceutical is administered orally. After giving the feed, the patient lies supine with a gamma camera positioned anteriorly over the chest and abdomen in the field of view. Any reflux of radiopharmaceutical into the oesophagus indicates the presence of GER.

Patient preparation: Nil per oral for 4 hours.

Radiopharmaceutical	**^{99m}Tc-Sulphur Colloid (SC)**
Route of administration	Oral or via NG tube (^{99m}Tc-SC mixed with milk, or 150 ml orange juice)
Dose	0.2-1.0 mCi (7.4-37 MBq)

Indications:

- Suspected GERD in neonates and in patients with GERD symptoms and negative UGI endoscopy.
- To confirm aspiration to lung (recurrent aspiration pneumonia).
- To look for reflux post TEF (tracheo-oesophageal fistula) repair.

Common imaging patterns

Normal milk scan

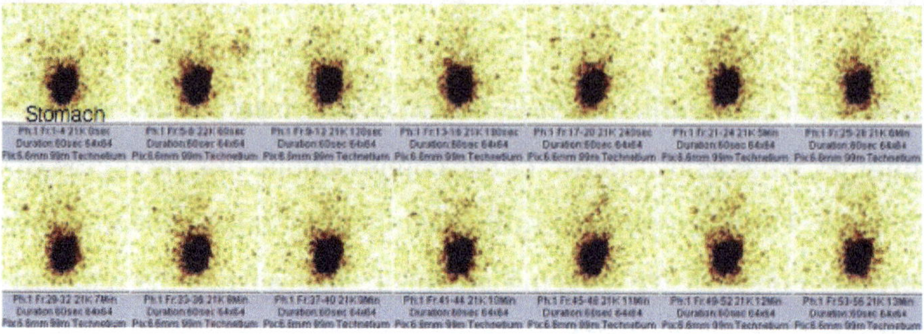

The tracer activity is seen in the stomach throughout the entire study with no reflux of contents into the oesophagus.

GERD: Oesophagus will be visualized due to the reflux of contents into the oesophagus. Reflux can be graded as below:

- **Low-grade** – Reflux into the lower one-third of oesophagus or reflux persisting for less than 10 seconds during the entire study.
- **High-grade** – Reflux reaching upto mid/upper third of oesophagus or reflux persisting for more than 10 seconds during the entire study.

Delayed lung images can be taken after 2 hours to evaluate **aspiration pneumonia**.

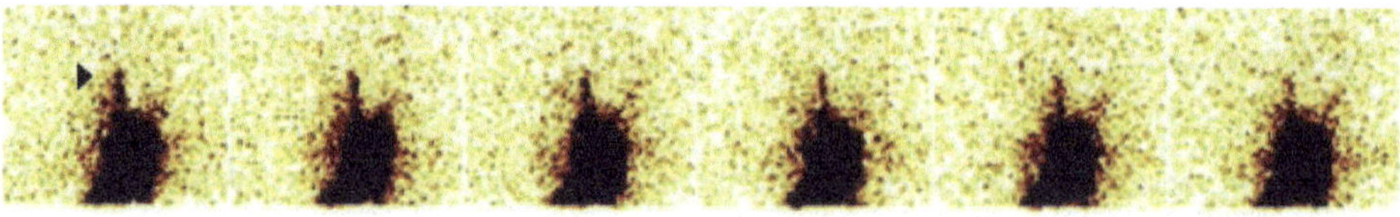

Persistent reflux of gastric contents up to the mid-third of the oesophagus in the above image, indicating high-grade GERD.

5.2 Gastric Emptying Time Scintigraphy

Radionuclide gastric emptying time (GET) study is a quantitative method to assess the rate of emptying of meal from the stomach. Gastric emptying can be either delayed or rapid in different diseases. Delayed gastric emptying is seen more commonly than rapid emptying, and the patient presents with early satiety, nausea, vomiting and bloating.

Patient preparation: Nil per oral for 4 hours. Fasting blood sugar should be less than 200 mg/dL. History of prokinetic drug intake should be recorded.

Radiopharmaceutical	**^{99m}Tc – Sulphur colloid labelled meal**
Route of administration	Oral (in a standard meal) followed by image acquisition upto 4 hours.
Dose (for adults)	1-2 mCi (37-74 MBq)

Types:

- Solid gastric emptying (assessed using solid meal).
- Liquid gastric emptying (assessed using liquid meal).

Indications:

- Gastroparesis in diabetic patients
- Dyspepsia symptoms
- Unexplained abdominal pain
- Assess response to a motility drug

Common imaging patterns

Normal GET study: After a standard solid meal, >10% gastric emptying at 1 hour, >40% at 2 hours and >90% at 4 hours after a standard solid meal.

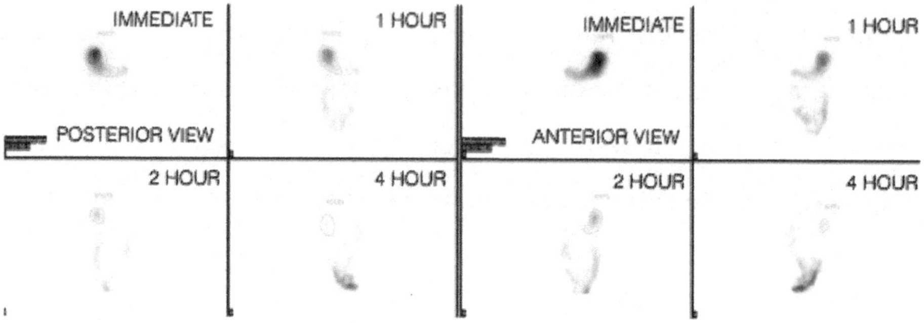

Anterior and posterior images of the stomach acquired at baseline, 1, 2 and 4 hours are seen. Region of interest (ROI) is drawn on the stomach and the percentage emptying at 1, 2 and 4 hours were found to be 52%, 85% and 99%, indicating a normal GET for a solid meal.

Abnormal gastric emptying study:

- **Rapid GET** - >70% gastric emptying at 1 hour.
- **Delayed GET**- Gastric emptying less than normal values.

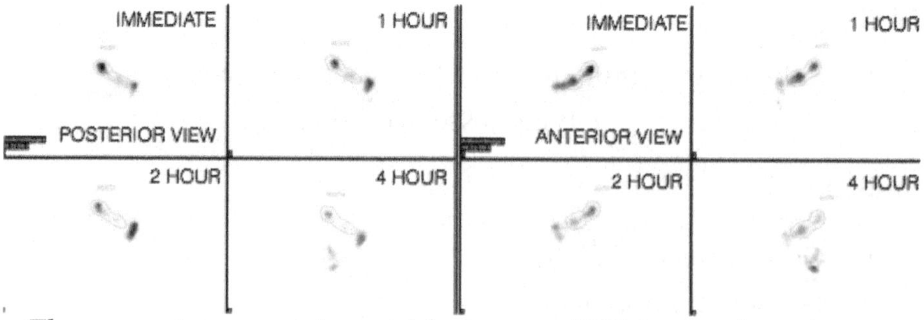

The percentage emptying at 4 hours was 59% in the above images, indicating delayed gastric emptying for a solid meal.

5.3 Gastrointestinal Bleed Scintigraphy

Mechanism: The radiopharmaceutical should remain within the blood pool and leak at the bleeding site. There should be low background activity in the abdomen with no physiological gastrointestinal uptake.

Patient preparation: No special preparation needed. Avoid imaging during blood transfusion. Perchlorate should be given orally before ^{99m}Tc-Red blood cell scan to block free pertechnetate uptake in the stomach.

Radiopharmaceutical	**^{99m}Tc-Red Blood Cell**	**^{99m}Tc-Sulphur Colloid**
Administration	Intravenous	Intravenous
Dose (for adults)	15-20 mCi (555-740 MBq)	2 mCi (74 MBq)

mCi, Millicurie; MBq, Mega Becquerel.

Indications

- To detect and localize the site of occult lower gastrointestinal bleeding;
    - Intermittent gastrointestinal bleed (particularly useful).
    - In cases with negative CT angiography or contra-indications to contrast administration.
- Risk stratification and to direct further intervention;
    - Positive scan - Active intervention.
    - Negative scan –Conservative management (reduces the rate of negative invasive angiograms in 20-50% cases).

Imaging patterns	
Normal ^{99m}Tc-Red Blood Cell Scintigraphy **(Negative for GI bleed)** • *Physiological tracer distribution is seen in blood pool in heart, spleen, liver, and major vessels.* • *No abnormal focal tracer uptake in rest of abdomen and pelvis.*	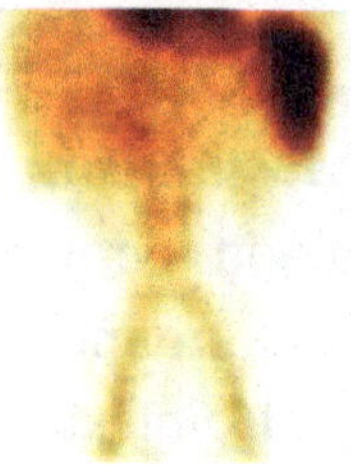
Positive ^{99m}Tc-Red Blood Cell Scintigraphy • *The focus of extravascular activity should start in a region where there was no abnormal activity before.* • *It should increase in intensity over time.* • *Should move either anterograde or retrograde fashion.* • *Should conform* to the contour of the bowel. • SPECT-CT can provide better anatomical localisation.	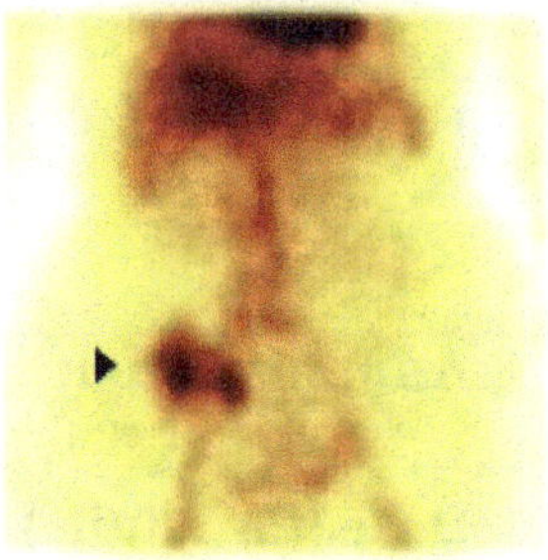

^{99m}Tc-Red blood cell scintigraphy is more sensitive than ^{99m}Tc-Sulphur colloid scintigraphy, particularly for intermittent bleeding. False positive interpretation can occur due to free Pertechnetate (gastric activity seen), uterine activity, ovulation, penile activity or focal vascular abnormalities without active bleed (e.g., aneurysms, splenosis, etc.).

5.4 Meckel Scintigraphy

Mechanism:

- Radiopharmaceutical concentrates in ectopic functioning gastric mucosa present in Meckel diverticulum via sodium iodide symporter (NIS).
- NIS expression has been reported in mucin-secreting cells and parietal cells in gastric mucosa.

Patient preparation: Fasting (4-6 hrs.). No barium study in last 3 days.

Radiopharmaceutical	**^{99m}Tc-Pertechnetate**
Administration	Intravenous
Dose (for adults)	0.05 mCi (1.85 MBq)/kg Minimum dose 1 mCi (37 MBq)

mCi, Millicurie; MBq, Mega Becquerel.

Indications:

- In children:
    - To detect Meckel's diverticulum in symptomatic cases with high clinical suspicion.
- To localize heterotopic gastric mucosa in:
        - Gastro-enteric duplication cyst.

- Retained gastric antrum after Billroth II gastrojejunostomy.
- Barrett'soesophagus.

Imaging patterns	
Normal scan • *Normal radiotracer uptake is seen in gastric mucosa.* • *Background blood pool and renal excretory activity is seen in the abdomen and pelvis.* • *No abnormal focal tracer uptake in rest of abdomen and pelvis.*	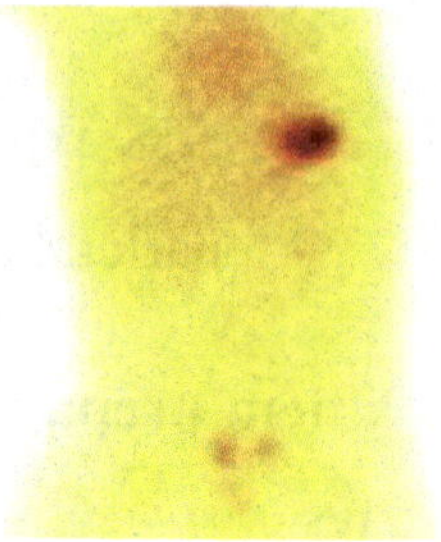
Meckel's diverticulum • *The activity appears at the same time in both normal stomach and ectopic mucosa (typically within 5-10 min in the right lower quadrant).* • *Increase in the tracer uptake over time (similar to the stomach).*	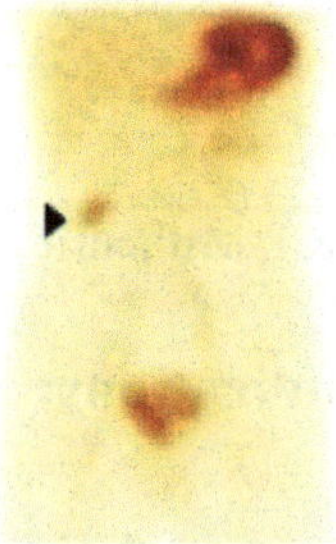

False negative results can occur due to small diverticula, impaired diverticular blood supply and recent barium study. False positive interpretation can occur due to urinary tract activity, vascular abnormalities, neoplasm, intussusception or volvulus.

5.5 Hepatobiliary Scintigraphy

Mechanism:

- ^{99m}Tc-Mebrofenin is an imino diacetic acid (IDA) derivative. It is an organic anion that binds to plasma proteins after intravenous injection and is extracted by the hepatocytes in a similar fashion to bilirubin, followed by excretion via the biliary system into the intestine, without undergoing metabolism or conjugation.
- Popularly known as Hepatobiliary IDA (HIDA) scan.

Patient preparation:

- Fasting 4 – 6 hours (avoid prolonged fasting).
- Opioids must be withheld for 6 hours before the scan.
- If the scan is done to rule out Extra Hepatic Biliary Atresia (EHBA), the child should be given Ursodeoxycholic acid (UDCA) 20 mg/kg/day or phenobarbitone 5mg/kg/day to induce liver enzymes for five days before the scan.

Radiopharmaceutical	**^{99m}Tc – Mebrofenin**
Administration	Intravenous
Dose (for adults)	4 mCi (148 MBq)
Dose (for children)	0.05 mCi (1.85 MBq/kg)

mCi, Millicurie;MBq, Mega Becquerel.

Indications

- In children:
    - To rule out EHBA and follow up after portoenterostomy.
    - Adjunct in the diagnosis of choledochal cyst.
- In adults:
    - Acute or chronic cholecystitis.
    - Sphincter of Oddi dysfunction.
    - Biliary leak assessment.
    - To assess the contractile function of the gall bladder using fatty meal stimulation/cholecystokinin.
    - Enterogastric reflux.

Common imaging patterns

1. Normal HIDA scan in a neonate:

When liver (hepatocyte) function is preserved, ^{99m}Tc-Mebrofenin will be extracted from the blood pool in 5 to 10 minutes and taken up by the liver.

The common bile duct and gall bladder will be well visualized by 20 and 30 minutes, respectively, after which the activity will be seen in the intestines. Visualization of intestinal activity indicates patent bilio-enteric drainage.

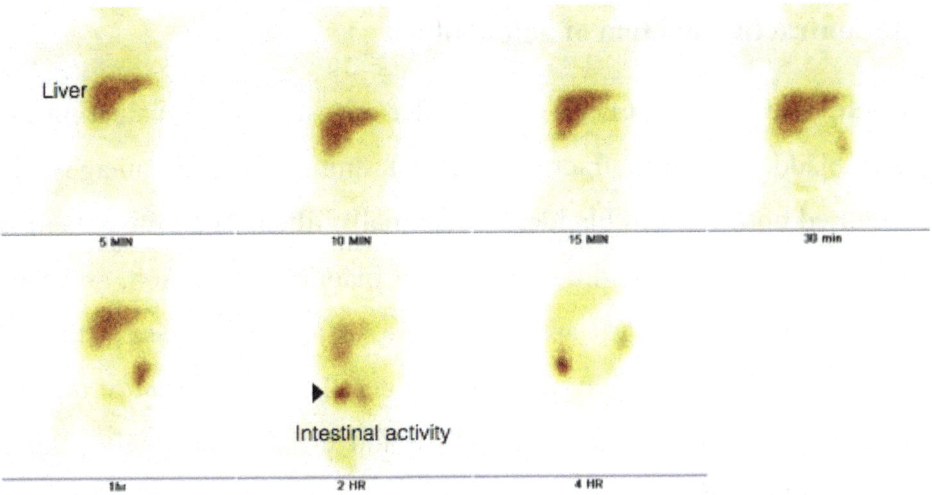

In the above image, both lobes of the liver show good hepatocyte tracer extraction (indicating good function) and visualization of the small intestinal loops by 30 minutes, confirming patent bilio-enteric drainage, hence ruling out EHBA.

2. EHBA

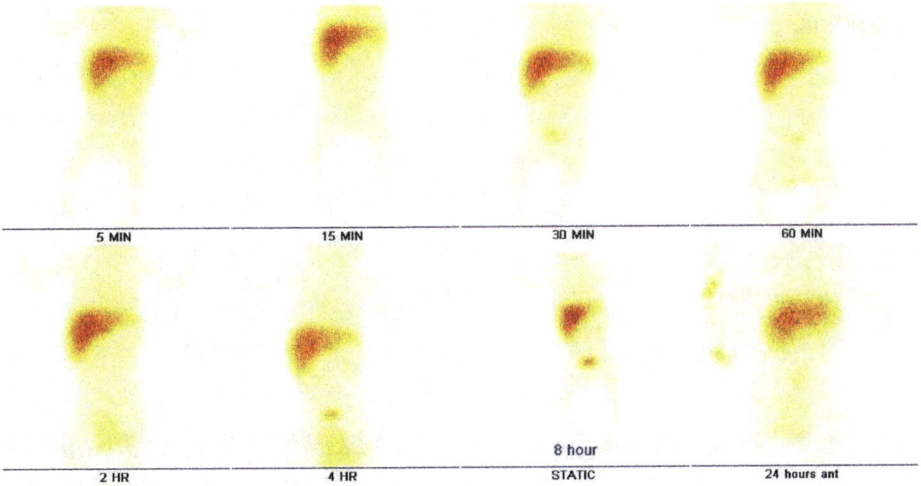

In the above image, both lobes of the liver show adequate hepatocyte tracer extraction (indicating good function), but no tracer activity is visualized in the intestinal loops till 24 hours and excretion of the tracer via kidney is seen. These findings are suggestive of EHBA.

3. Contractile function of gall bladder

Contractile function of the gall bladder is assessed by evaluating the gall bladder ejection fraction (GBEF). Initial dynamic images are acquired until the gall bladder is maximally filled. Then the patient is given a fatty meal to stimulate the gall bladder contraction, and then post-meal static images are acquired to evaluate the percentage of ejection of the tracer from the gall bladder. The lower limit of normal GBEF at 30 and 60 minutes is 27% and 60%, respectively after a standard fatty meal.

Impaired GB contractility:

If the gall bladder contraction is impaired, the GBEF values will be lower than the normal limit. GB contractility can be impaired secondary to drugs and multiple diseases, including diabetes, cirrhosis, etc.

The above image shows the maximal gall bladder filling at 30 minutes of the study (left panel) and the post-meal image acquired after one-hour (right panel), shows normal GB emptying (GBEF 90%).

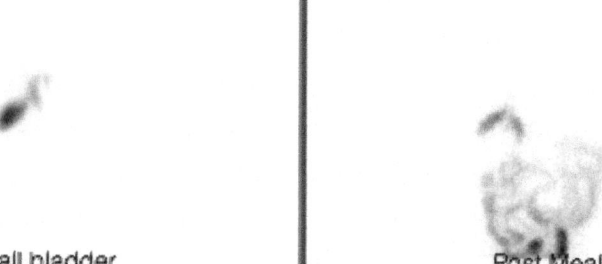

4. Biliary leak

Biliary leak can be post-traumatic or iatrogenic. HIDA scan is helpful to assess the presence of an active bile leak and identify the possible site. A rapid active leak is significant, requiring urgent management, while a slow leak is managed conservatively. There will be no abnormal tracer collection outside the bilio-enteric system in a patient with no biliary leak. If there is an abnormal collection of tracer activity outside the normal path of bilio-enteric drainage, it indicates a biliary leak.

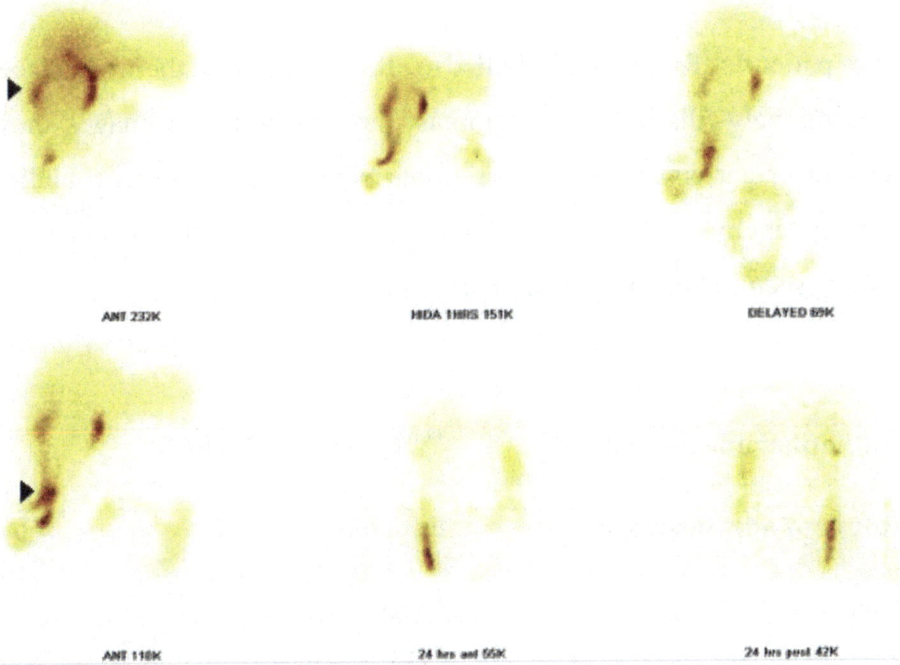

In the above image, abnormal focus of tracer activity is seen along the right lateral surface of the liver, which is seen to track down to the sub-hepatic space. These findings suggest an active bile leak.

5.6 Liver Blood Pool Scan

Cavernous hemangioma is the most common benign tumour of the liver. Usually, they are solitary, but sometimes there can be multiple hemangiomas in the liver. Liver blood pool scan using ^{99m}Tc-labelled red blood Cells (RBC) helps in the non-invasive diagnosis of liver hemangiomas.

Mechanism:

The patient's RBCs are labelled with ^{99m}Tc, and the radiotracer progressively fills into hemangiomas. Initial blood pool images show low tracer activity in the hemangioma compared to the surrounding liver parenchyma. With progressive filling, increased tracer activity will be seen in hemangiomas in later images.

Radiopharmaceutical	**^{99m}Tc–labelled RBCs**
Route of administration	Intravenous
Dose (for adults)	15-20 mCi (555-740 MBq)

mCi, Millicurie;MBq, Mega Becquerel.

Indication: To confirm suspected hemangiomas of the liver and other soft tissue organs.

Imaging pattern

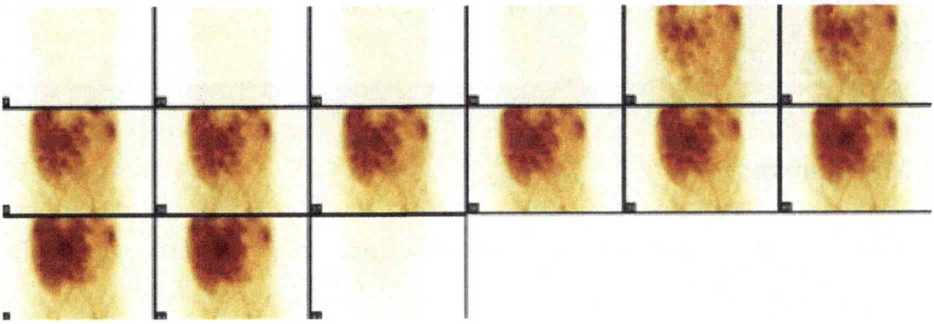

^{99m}Tc-labelled RBC liver scan showing progressive accumulation of tracer in the suspected liver lesions. This finding is suggestive of hemangiomas in the liver.

5.7 Liver-Spleen Scan

Mechanism:

^{99m}Tc-sulphur colloid is phagocytosed by cells of the reticuloendothelial system:

- Kupffer cells of the liver (85%);
- Macrophages of the spleen (10%);
- Bone marrow (5%).

Radiopharmaceutical	**^{99m}Tc – Sulphur Colloid**
Route of administration	Intravenous
Dose (for adults)	4 mCi (148 MBq)

mCi, Millicurie;MBq, Mega Becquerel.

Indications:

- To differentiate cirrhosis and non-cirrhotic portal fibrosis (NCPF).
- To differentiate focal nodular hyperplasia (FNH) from other liver lesions.
- To identify functioning splenic tissue and splenosis, e.g. in idiopathic thrombocytopenic purpura before splenectomy.

Imaging procedure: Twenty minutes after intravenous injection of ^{99m}Tc-sulphur colloid, planar static images of the liver and spleen are obtained.

Common imaging patterns

Cirrhosis of the liver and NCPF may have a similar clinical presentation; liver-spleen scan can assist in differentiating the two.

Cirrhosis:

Liver cirrhosis affects both hepatocytes and Kupffer cells similarly, which results in decreased tracer uptake in the liver due to the destruction of Kupffer cells. In cirrhotic liver disease, increased tracer uptake is seen in the spleen and bone marrow due to the shift of tracer to these organs, known as *colloid shift.*

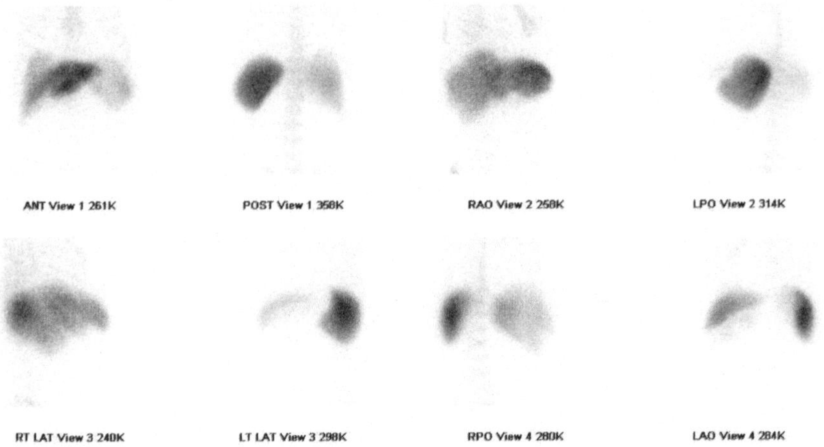

Impaired hepatocyte function and increased tracer uptake seen in spleen and bone marrow indicating colloid shift, favouring cirrhosis.

Non-cirrhotic portal fibrosis:

NCPF is characterized by fibrosis of small and medium branches of the portal vein, but the liver structure and function remain normal.

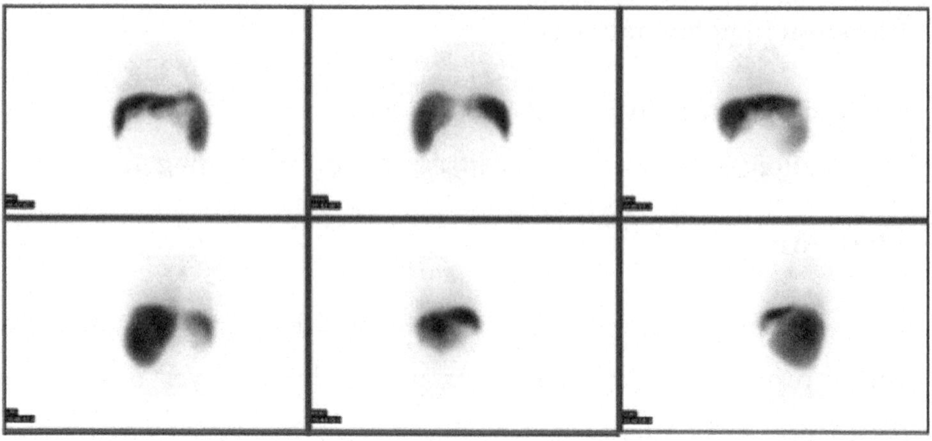

In the above image, the hepatocyte function is preserved, and there is no evidence of a colloid shift, suggestive of NCPF.

Section 6

Nuclear Cardiology

Dr. TK Nitheesh Raj

Dr. Anwin Joseph K

Dr. Harpreet Singh

Dr. Ashwani Sood

6.1 Myocardial Perfusion Imaging (MPI)

Introduction: Myocardial perfusion imaging (MPI) is the most commonly done procedure in Nuclear Cardiology. Radiotracers, which are taken up by the cardiac myocytes (myocardium) in linear relation to the blood flow are injected to assess regional myocardial perfusion at peak stress and/or rest. Single photon emission computed tomography (SPECT) images of the cardiac region are acquired in gating mode, reconstructed and processed to obtain perfusion images of the left ventricular (LV) myocardium.

Radiopharmaceutical	^{201}Thallous Chloride	^{99m}Tc-Sestamibi	^{99m}Tc-Tetrofosmin
Half-life	73 hours	6 hours	6 hours
Photon energy	69-81,167 keV	140 keV	140 keV
First pass extraction	~85%	~65%	~55%
Excretion	Renal	Hepatobiliary	Hepatobiliary
Mechanism of uptake	Sodium potassium ATPase	Passive diffusion (localise to mitochondria)	Similar to ^{99m}Tc-sestamibi
Dose	3 mCi (111 MBq)	10-30 mCi (370-1110 MBq)	10-30 mCi (370-1110 MBq)

Imaging time after tracer injection	10 min. after stress with redistribution image after 3 hours.	15-30 min. after stress. 30-90 min. after rest.	5-15 min. after stress and 30 min. after rest injection.

mCi, Millicurie;MBq, Mega Becquerel.

Stress Protocol

Stress myocardial perfusion imaging is done to assess the presence of ischemia. Exercise stress can be done using treadmill or bicycle ergometer. Exercise using a treadmill is done according to the standardized protocols (most often the Bruce or modified Bruce protocol) with incremental treadmill speed and incline. Pharmacological stress is used when exercise stress is contraindicated/cannot be performed or where exercise can lead to false-positive findings.

The principle behind Stress MPI

Physical exercise increases the cardiac workload, which in turn increases the myocardial oxygen demand. Normal coronary arteries dilate to meet the increased oxygen demand of the myocardium. Coronary vessels with flow-limiting stenosis cannot dilate further leading to less delivery and localisation of the radiopharmaceutical to the myocardium supplied by the stenotic coronary artery, which is seen as a relative perfusion defect (area of reduced tracer uptake surrounded by adjacent non-ischemic myocardium with normal perfusion/ tracer uptake).

Indications of Stress MPI

1. To diagnose obstructive coronary artery disease (CAD) in patients with an intermediate pre-test probability of CAD, Diabetes mellitus and in patients considered CAD equivalents (i.e. patients with chronic kidney disease or peripheral vascular disease).
2. Risk stratification of post-myocardial infarction (MI) patients.
3. Risk stratification of patients with chronic stable angina to guide therapy (medical management vs coronary revascularization).
4. Risk stratification before major noncardiac surgery in known/high risk CAD patients (e.g. before renal/liver transplant).
5. To evaluate the therapeutic efficacy of anti-ischemic medicines or coronary revascularization.
6. Cardiac mechanical dyssynchrony assessment.

Basic interpretation:

- Images are displayed as slices along the short axis, vertical long axis and horizontal long axis of the LV myocardium.
- If a perfusion defect is present on stress images, which normalizes on rest images, it indicates ischemic myocardium.
- If a significant perfusion defect is present on both the stress and rest images, it indicates an infarct/scar.
- Cardiac wall motion, volumes, ejection fraction and dyssynchrony can also be assessed using gated MPI SPECT.

Patient preparation for exercise stress:

- Fasting for 4 hours.
- Beta-blockers, calcium channel blockers and nitrates should be discontinued for at least 24-48 hours before the study (or until 4-6 half-lives of the drug).
- The patient should wear loose clothes and sports shoes on the day of the test.
- A 24G IV line should be placed (for radiotracer administration).

Contraindications for Exercise stress:

- High-risk unstable angina.
- Decompensated heart failure.
- Cardiac arrhythmias causing hemodynamic compromise.
- Uncontrolled hypertension >200/110 mmHg.
- Acute pulmonary embolism/ severe pulmonary hypertension.
- Acute MI.
- Severe aortic stenosis.
- Acute aortic dissection.

Exercise stress

- Electrocardiogram, blood pressure and pulse should be continuously monitored during the stress and recovery period.
- The endpoint should be symptom limited (like chest pain and breathlessness). The achievement of 85% of the maximum predicted heart rate for exercise stress is not an indication for termination of stress.

- The radiopharmaceutical is injected during the peak of the exercise, and the exercise is continued further for atleast 1 minute following radiotracer administration.

Indications for early termination of stress:

- Moderate to severe angina or dyspnoea.
- Excessive fatigue.
- Ataxia, dizziness and syncope.
- Significant ST-segment depression or elevation.
- Drop in systolic BP >10mmHg from baseline.
- Significant rise in BP > 230/ 115mmHg.
- Sustained supraventricular and ventricular tachycardia.
- Patients request to terminate.

Pharmacological stress can be done using vasodilators or Dobutamine (inotropic action, increases cardiac contractility). Pharmacological stress is used when exercise stress is contraindicated, cannot be performed or where exercise can lead to false-positive findings.

Vasodilator stress agents

	Adenosine	Dipyridamole	Regadenoson
Mechanism of action	Direct coronary arteriolar vasodilation through activation of the Adenosine 2A (A2A) receptors	Indirect coronary dilator, whichinhibits the reuptake of adenosine	Adenosine analogue with high affinity towards A2A receptors
Dose	140 μg/kg/min i.v. infusion for 6 minutes	0.56 mg/kg i.v. Infusion for 4 minutes	0.4 mg bolus
Timing of tracer injection	At 3 min. of infusion	3-5 min after the completion of infusion.	20-30 seconds after bolus injection

Patient preparation for vasodilator stress:

- Avoid caffeinated drinks 12-24 hours before the test.
- Methylxanthines should be stopped for 24-48 hours.

Side effects: Minor side effects like chest pain, dyspnoea, dizziness, nausea and symptomatic hypotension can occur. Rare side effects include atrioventricular blocks, ST-segment depression, MI, and atrial fibrillation.

MPI Image

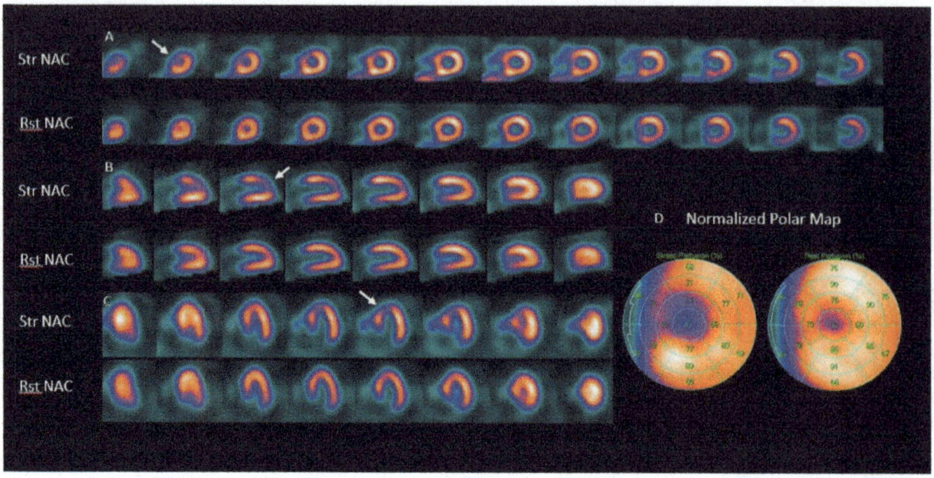

Stress (Str)-rest (Rst) myocardial perfusion images in short axis (A), vertical long axis (B) and horizontal long axis (C) demonstrates a reversible perfusion defect (arrows) in the distal anteroseptal wall [Left anterior descending artery territory]. Polar map display (D) of left ventricular radiotracer distribution during stress and rest (Bright areas denote normal perfusion while dark areas denote reduced perfusion).

6.2 Equilibrium Radionuclide Angiography (ERNA)

Equilibrium Radionuclide Angiography (ERNA):

- Also known as MUGA (multi-gated acquisition) study and Radionuclide Ventriculography.
- ERNA is used for the assessment of global and regional ventricular function.

Mechanism:

- First pass study is done to assess the initial transit of tracer through circulation and right ventricular (RV) function.
- Equilibrium blood pool study (ERNA) is used to assess cardiac function over multiple cardiac cycles (mainly LV function). ERNA is done by labelling of RBC's with ^{99m}Tc-pertechnetate.
- Three main methods of RBC labelling are in vivo, in vitro (97% labelling efficiency) and modified in vivo (85% labelling efficiency) methods.

Radiopharmaceutical	**^{99m}Tc – RBC**
Administration	Intravenous
Dose (for adults)	15-20 mCi (555-740 MBq)

mCi, Millicurie;MBq, Mega Becquerel.

Indications:

- Assessment of LV function.

- Assessment of anthracycline-induced cardiotoxicity;
    - Assessment of LV function at baseline and sequential follow up.
    - Discontinue cardiotoxic therapy if >10% decrease in LV ejection fraction (EF) to value of less than 50%.
- Assessment of coronary artery disease.
- To differentiate pulmonary vs. LV cause of RV enlargement.
- Congenital heart disease – assessment of right-left shunt.
- Assessment of LV dyssynchrony.
- Assessment of diastolic dysfunction in patients with heart failure.

Advantages:

- Non-invasive modality, less operator dependence, high reproducibility, and easy to perform, even in sick patients.
- Accurate LVEF calculations because LV counts are proportional to LV volume over the cardiac cycle.

Disadvantages:

- Prone to errors in case of heart rate variability or arrhythmias (Prevalence of >10% premature ventricular contractions).

Patient preparation/ pre-requisites:

- Electrocardiogram to confirm the normal sinus rhythm of the patient.

Contra-indications: None.

Procedure (with modified in vivo method): After confirming normal sinus rhythm, inject reducing agent (stannous chloride 15 μgm/kg) intravenously, followed by ^{99m}Tc-pertechnetate injection after 20 minutes. Imaging is done after 10-15 minutes.

Findings:

- Images are reviewed and processed using software to obtain different functional parameters:
  - Size, position and rotation of heart and great vessels.
  - Chamber sizes of atria and ventricles.
  - Global and regional LVEF (Normal global LVEF >50%).
  - Global and regional wall motion.
  - Peak filling rates of ventricles.

Blood pool SPECT MUGA can also be done for 3-dimensional imaging. In addition, multiple functional images are obtained:

- **Stroke volume (SV) image** by pixel-wise subtraction of end-systolic (ES) from end-diastolic (ED) image, which reflects regional stroke volume in ml.
- **Ejection fraction (EF) image** by pixel-wise division of SV image from ED volume.
- **Paradox image** by subtracting ED from ES image (highlights areas of paradoxical ventricular wall motion).
- **Amplitude image** denotes the amplitude of cardiac contractility.
- **Phase analysis image** gives measures of dyssynchrony (Peak phase, phase standard deviation, histogram bandwidth, histogram skewness (asymmetry) and histogram kurtosis).

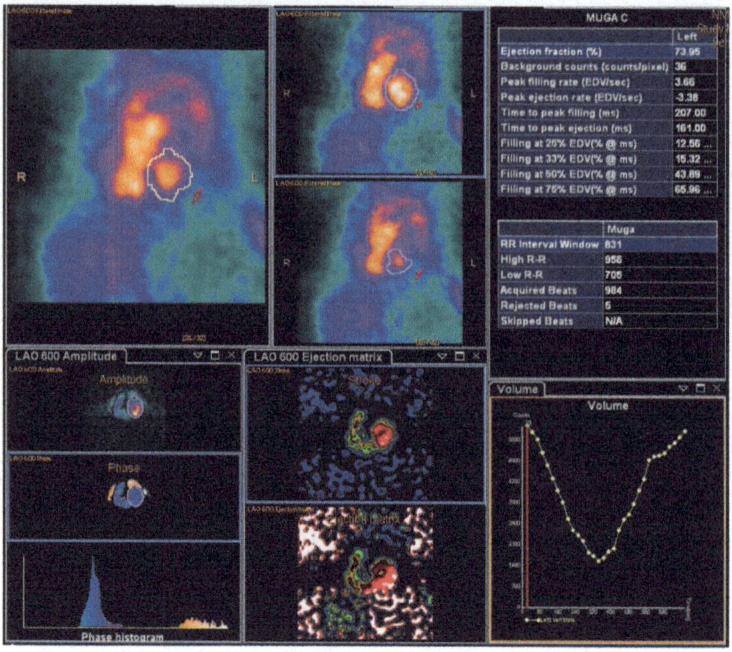

Normal MUGA scan (Normal sized LV cavity and LVEF)

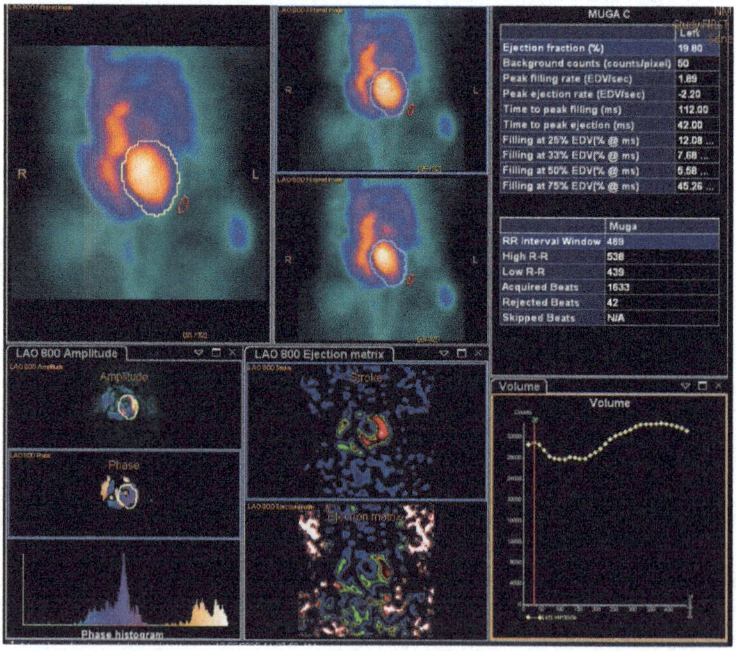

Dilated left ventricular cavity with reduced LVEF (20%) on MUGA.

6.3 Myocardial Viability & Flow Reserve

Myocardial viability assessment using PET

Mechanism:

- Hibernating myocardium is the viable but dysfunctional myocardium due to compromised regional blood flow, identification and revascularization of which can lead to improvement in the myocardial function.
- Myocardium uses glucose and fatty acid as fuel sources. Oral glucose loading combined with intravenous insulin can increase the probability of glucose being used as the source of energy by the viable myocardium.
- Perfusion can be assessed using various PET or SPECT perfusion tracers and metabolism using ^{18}F-FDG, which is a glucose analogue PET tracer.

PET perfusion agents

Radiopharmaceutical	Half-life	Production method
^{82}Rb-RbCl	76 sec.	^{82}Sr – ^{82}Rb generator
^{13}N-ammonia	10 min.	Cyclotron
^{18}F-flupiridaz	110 min.	Cyclotron
^{15}O-water	2 min.	Cyclotron

SPECT perfusion agents:

- ^{99m}Tc-sestamibi/tetrofosmin MPI (Rest study with nitrate augmentation can be done)
- ^{201}Thallous chloride MPI (rest-redistribution study)

PET metabolic agent

Radiopharmaceutical	Half-life	Production
^{18}F-FDG	110 min.	Cyclotron

Indication:

Patients with CAD, LV dysfunction and having resting myocardial perfusion defects to differentiate viable (hibernating) vs. non-viable (scar) myocardium and decide whether coronary revascularisation will be beneficial or not.

Patient Preparation and Procedure

Procedure	Steps
Preparation	Fasting 6-12 hours
Rest perfusion study	**SPECT** tracers: (see *section 6.1*), or, **PET** tracers: ^{13}N-ammonia-15-20 mCi (550-740 MBq) or ^{82}Rb-Rubidium chloride 30 mCi (1100 MBq)
^{18}F-FDG PET	**Glucose loading** Fasting blood glucose (FBG) is checked and

	glucose load 25-100 gram orally is given if FBG<250 mg/dL. Glucose loading is not necessary if FBG>250 mg/dL. Blood glucose is checked after 45-60 minutes. Regular insulin is administered i.v. and monitoring is done till blood glucose level falls to <150 mg/dL.
^{18}F-FDG Injection	5-10 mCi (185-370 MBq) ^{18}F-FDG
Imaging	Imaging 45-60 minutes after ^{18}F-FDG injection. In diabetic patients, imaging after 90-120 minutes may be more appropriate.

mCi, Millicurie;MBq, Mega Becquerel.

Basic interpretation:

- Normal LV perfusion on rest MPI indicates that the myocardium is viable (and further, ^{18}F-FDG PET imaging is not needed).
- Presence of metabolism in a segment of myocardium showing significant perfusion defect (mismatched defect), indicates that myocardium is viable (hibernating).
- Absence of metabolism in a segment of myocardium showing significant perfusion defect (matched defect), indicates that myocardium is non-viable (scar).

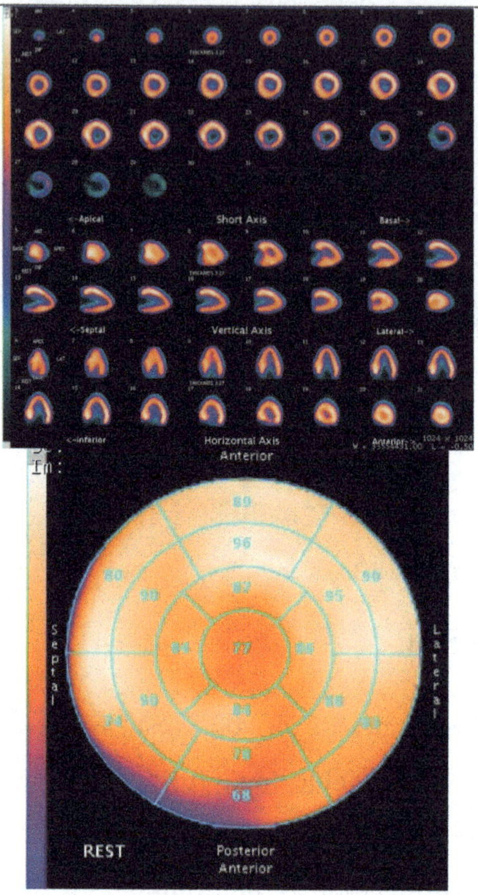

Normal perfusion

Left: $^{13}N\text{-}NH_3$ perfusion PET images in short axis (upper rows), vertical long axis (middle rows) and horizontal long axis (bottom rows) views showing adequate perfusion in all the walls of LV myocardium. Right: Polar plot image (2-D representation of the LV myocardium) showing adequate perfusion in all the segments of LV myocardium indicating viable LV myocardium.

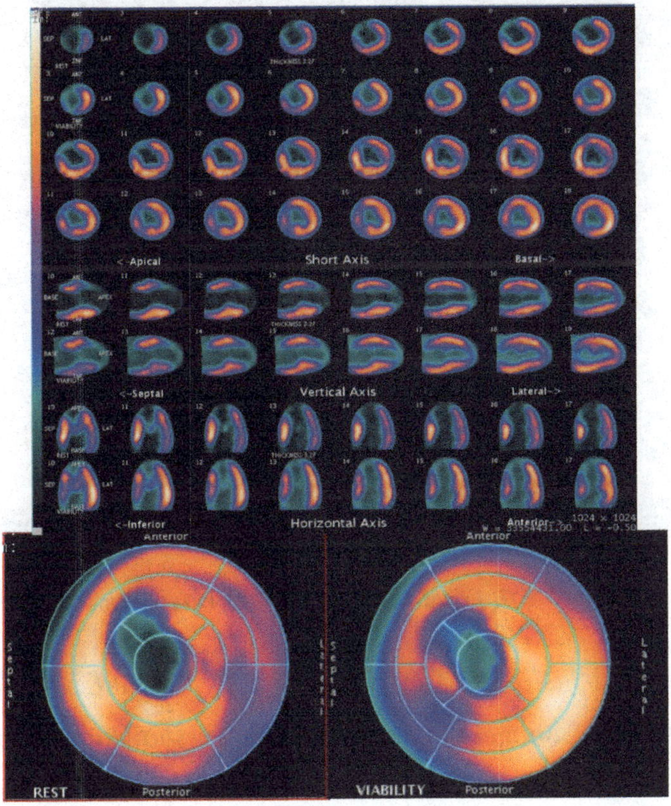

Perfusion-metabolism match

[13]N-NH3 perfusion PET images (rows: 1, 3, 5 and 7) and ^{18}F-FDG metabolic PET images (rows: 2, 4, 6 and 8) showing severely reduced perfusion and metabolism involving parts of mid and distal anterior wall, anteroseptal wall and apex of LV myocardium, suggestive of non-viable myocardium (LAD territory). Polar plot of perfusion (rest) and metabolism (viability) also demonstrating the same findings.

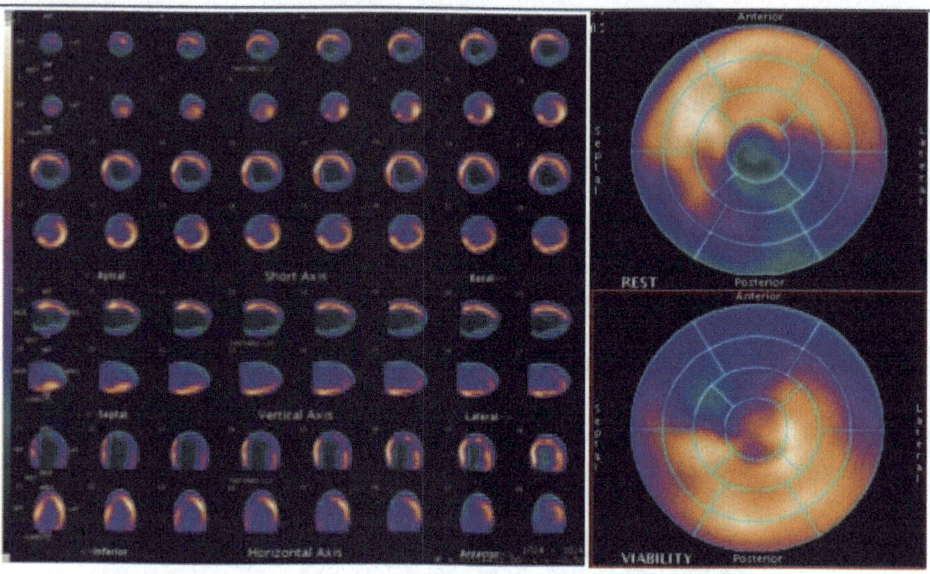

Perfusion-metabolism mismatch

^{13}N-NH_3 perfusion PET images (rows: 1, 3, 5 and 7) and ^{18}F-FDG metabolic PET images (rows: 2, 4, 6 and 8) showing severely reduced perfusion but adequate metabolism involving the inferior wall and adjacent parts of inferolateral and inferoseptal walls suggestive of hibernating but viable myocardium (Right coronary / left circumflex artery territory). Polar plot of perfusion (rest) and metabolism (viability) also demonstrating the same findings.

Myocardial flow reserve (MFR) estimation

Mechanism:

- Rest and stress dynamic PET perfusion images are acquired in list mode using modern PET scanners.
- Time-activity curves for the arterial blood and myocardial regions are used as inputs.
- The rate of tracer uptake in myocardial tissue provides an estimate of the absolute global and regional myocardial blood flow (MBF in mL/min/g). MBF at rest is coupled with myocardial oxygen demand. Normal resting MBF ranges from 0.4-1.2 ml/min/gram.
- The ratio of MBF at peak stress to rest gives the myocardial flow reserve (MFR). Earlier, called as coronary flow reserve (CFR).

Interpretation and uses:

- MFR >2 is associated with low risk of major adverse cardiac events while MFR <1.5 denotes higher risk of cardiac events and has higher sensitivity for early detection of CAD.
- Added value for detecting multivessel disease with balanced ischemia, which may be falsely negative on SPECT myocardial perfusion imaging.
  - Useful for detecting microvascular dysfunction.
  - Prognostic marker in CAD patients.

Common imaging patterns

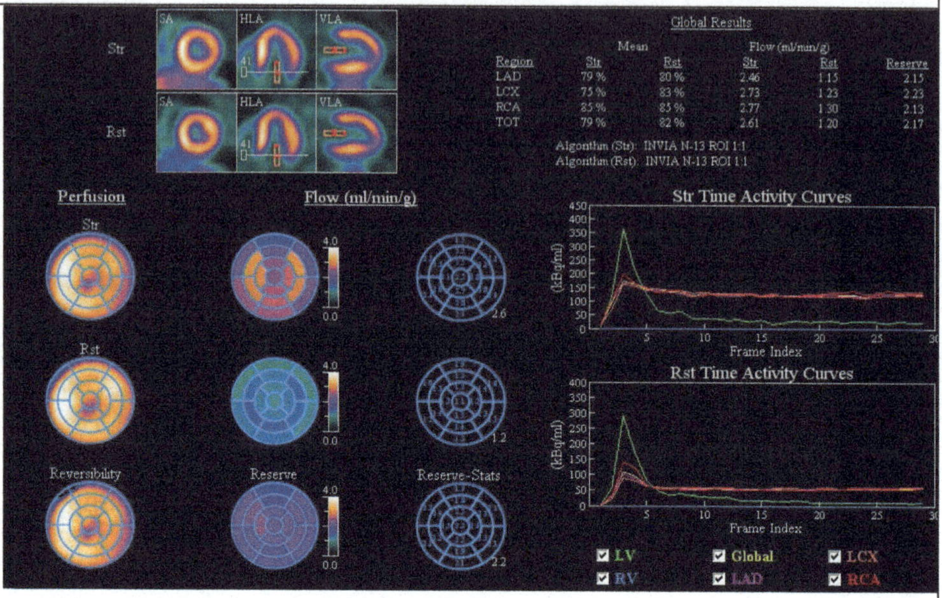

^{13}N-NH$_3$ cardiac PET: Cross-sectional and polar plot images of the stress and rest study depicting normal perfusion in all the segments of LV myocardium. The time-activity curves on the right side showing global and territorial normal MFR (>2.0).

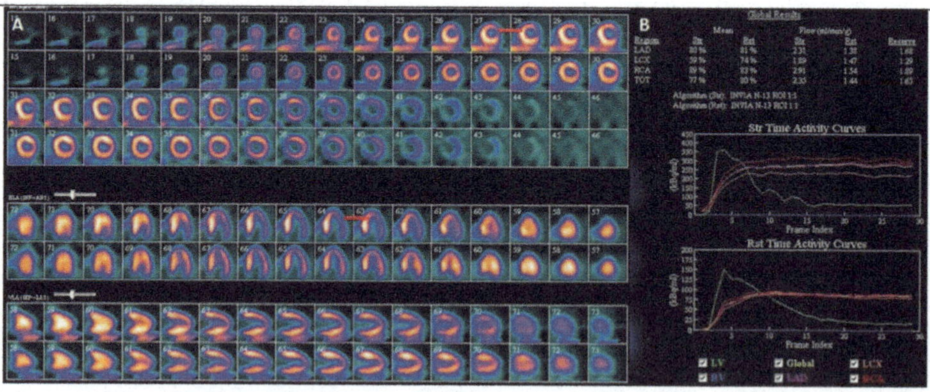

^{13}N-NH$_3$ cardiac PET: Cross sectional images depict a reversible perfusion defect in the anterolateral wall. The time-activity curves on the right side shows a reduction in global MFR 1.63 (< 2.0) with severe reduction in MFR (1.29) in left circumflex artery territory.

Section 7

Ventilation Perfusion (VQ) Scintigraphy

Dr. Abdul Waheed
Dr. Harmandeep Singh

7 Ventilation Perfusion (VQ) Scintigraphy

Mechanism: Ventilation agents are used to measure airflow distribution in the lung. Radiopharmaceuticals used as perfusion agents help to delineate the blood flow distribution in the bilateral lung fields. Perfusion agents contain particles ranging in size from 10 to 100 μm, which lodge in the pre-capillary arterioles in the lungs.

Patient preparation: No special preparation needed.

VENTILATION AGENTS are either aerosols (99mTc-DTPA/Technegas) or radioactive gases (Xenon-133/Krypton-81m).

Radiopharmaceutical	**^{99m}Tc -DTPA**	**Technegas**
Administration	Inhalation	Inhalation
Dose (for adults)	0.5-1.1 mCi (20-40 MBq)	0.5-0.8 mCi (20-30 MBq)

PERFUSION AGENTS

Radiopharmaceutical	**^{99m}Tc - Macro-aggregated albumin (MAA)**
Route	Intravenous
Dose	3-5 mCi (111-185 MBq) with 2-5 lakh particles

The number of particles to be injected is decreased in case of children younger than 5 years, patients with pulmonary hypertension, and right to left cardiac shunt.

Indications:

- To determine the likelihood of pulmonary embolism (PE).

Clinical scenarios in which VQ scan is appropriate for PE diagnosis

- PE-likely and D-dimer-Negative
- PE-likely and Chest X ray-normal or mildly abnormal
- PE-likely and abnormal RFT/contrast complications.
- PE-likely and CT pulmonary angiography finding-discordant

- Document resolution of PE.
- Measure differential pulmonary function before pulmonary surgery, in cases with congenital heart or lung disease.
- Assessment of lung transplants.
- Chronic pulmonary hypertension.

Technical considerations: ^{99m}Tc-MAA should be injected slowly over multiple respiratory cycles with patient in supine position. Blood should not be withdrawn into the syringe.

Interpretation:

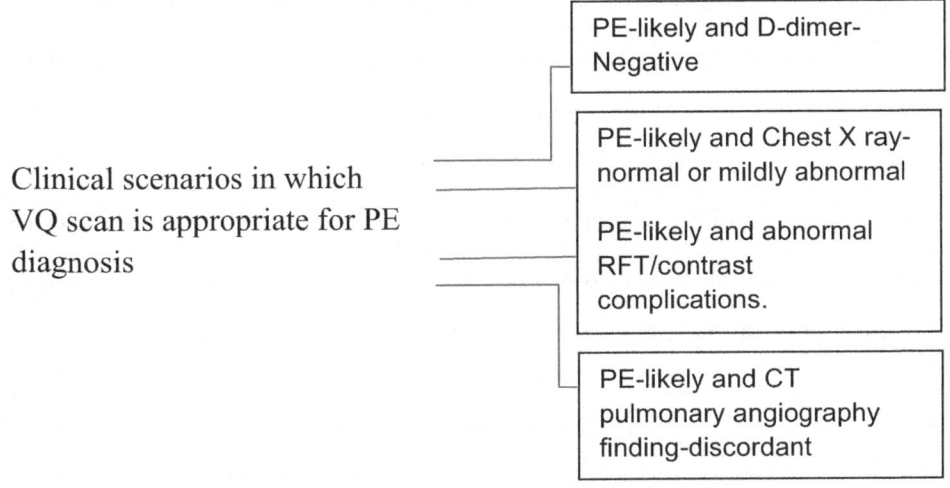

VQ scan may be performed as a planar or SPECT study. Ventilation scan findings need to be compared with perfusion scan. If ventilation scan is not available, comparison with X-ray chest or CT chest (in case of SPECT-CT) can be done. SPECT has increased diagnostic accuracy compared to planar imaging. Detection of sub-segmental defects and defects in medial segments of the lungs is better with SPECT.

Multiple criteria exist to interpret VQ scan and give probability of PE. Basic interpretation is based on presence of VQ mismatch (ventilation present, perfusion absent) in at least one pulmonary segment or two sub-segments (wedge-shaped defects with the base projecting to the lung periphery), which favours PE. On the other hand, VQ matched defect (Both ventilation and perfusion absent) or reverse-matched VQ defect, or any defect, which does not follow segmental anatomy, do not suggest PE.

Common imaging patterns

99mTc-MAA Lung perfusion scan

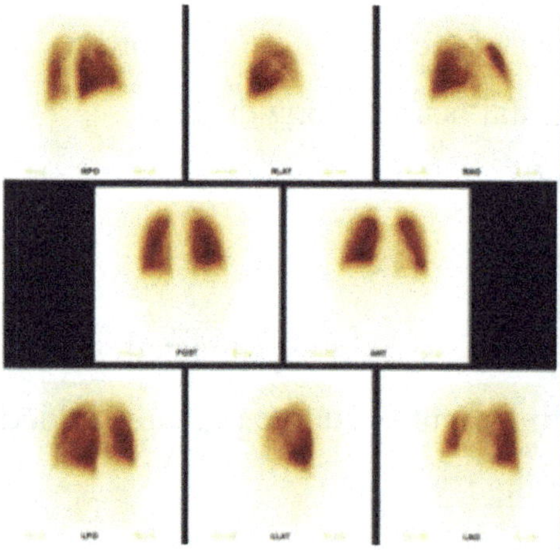

Normal lung perfusion scan.

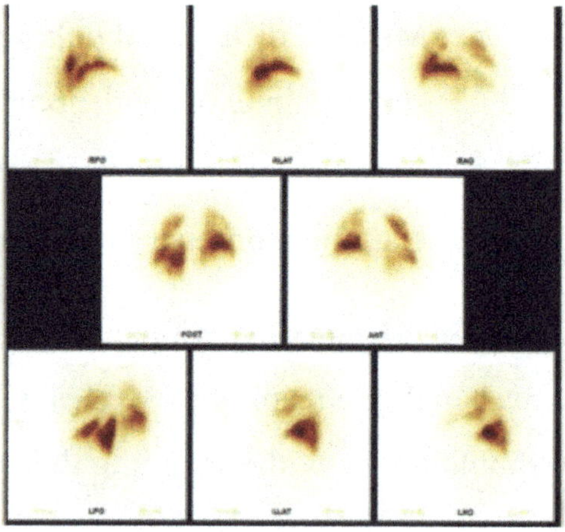

Multiple wedge-shaped segmental defects in bilateral lung fields on ^{99m}Tc-MAA scan, suggestive of pulmonary embolism.

VQ SPECT-CT		
Normal scan • *No perfusion defect on SPECT* • *Normal lung parenchyma on CT.*	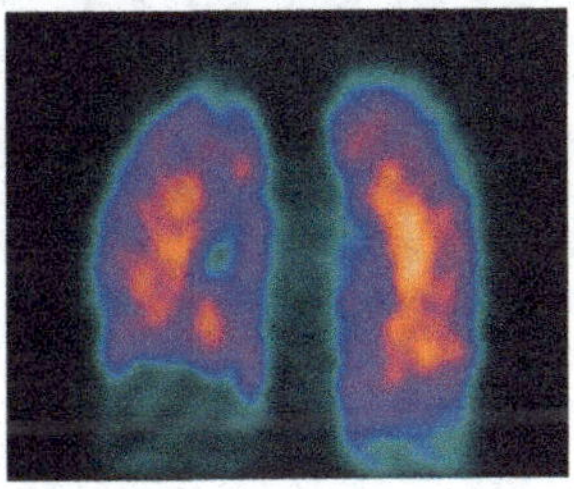	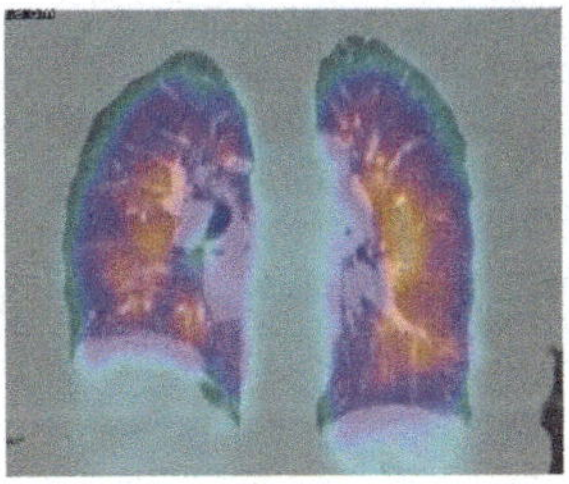
VQ Matched defect • *Perfusion defect on SPECT.* • *Lung parenchymal abnormality in corresponding area on CT.* • *Not suggestive of pulmonary embolism.*	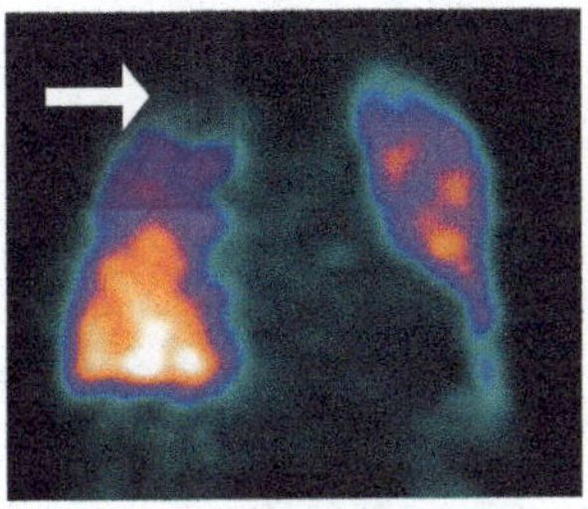 Right upper lobe defect	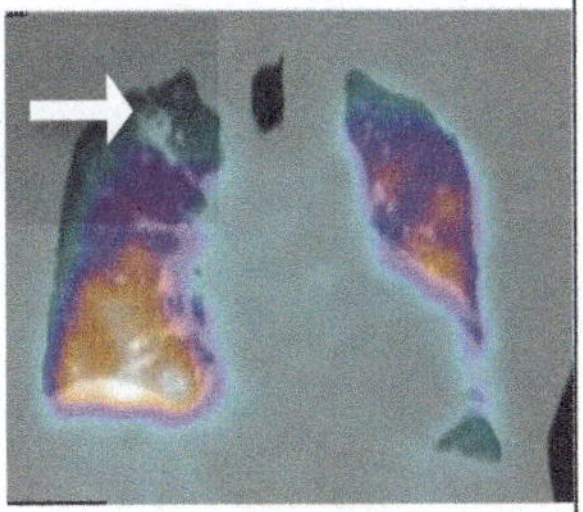 Fibrocalcific changes on CT
VQ Mismatched defect • *Wedge shaped perfusion defect on SPECT.* • *No abnormality in corresponding area on CT.* • *Segmental defect or multiple sub-segmental defects - suggestive of pulmonary embolism.*	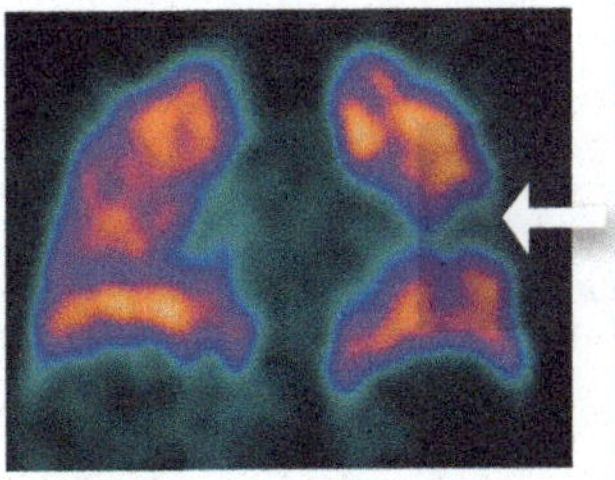 Segmental defect in lingula of left lung	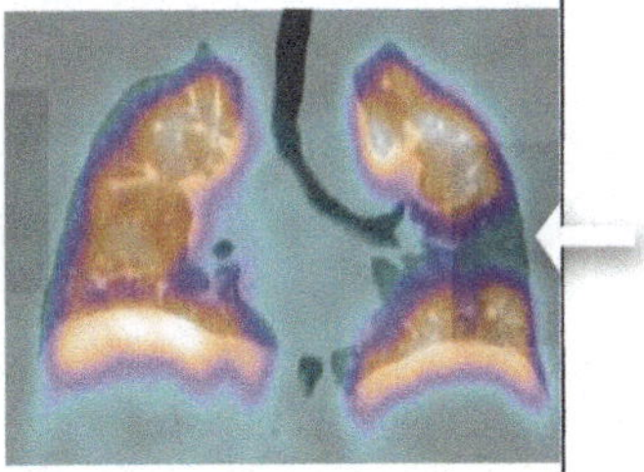 Normal lung parenchyma on CT

Section 8

Central Nervous System

Dr. Venkata Subramanian K

Dr. Harmandeep Singh

8.1 Central Nervous System

^{18}F–FDG PET/CT

- ^{18}F–FDG is a glucose analogue.
- Glucose accounts for 95% of energy consumption in brain.
- Brain metabolism is tightly coupled to perfusion and neuronal activity. 18F-FDG PET can identify areas of increased or decreased metabolism in the brain.

Radiopharmaceutical	**^{18}F- FDG**
Administration route	Intravenous
Radioactivity (Dose for adults)	4-5 mCi (148-185 MBq)

Indications:

- For differential diagnosis of dementia.
- For assessment of atypical Parkinson syndromes in patients presenting with movement disorders.
- For localization of epileptogenic focus in patients presenting with refractory focal seizures (both temporal and extra-temporal).
- For evaluation of CNS involvement in systemic pathologies (infective, inflammatory or neoplastic).

Common Imaging patterns

Normal ^{18}F-FDG Brain PET scan

- *Bilaterally symmetrical FDG uptake is seen in bilateral cerebral and cerebellar cortices, basal ganglia and thalami.*
- *Grey matter uptake is 2.5-4 times higher than the white matter uptake.*
- *Basal ganglia uptake is higher than neocortex.*
- *Visual, posterior cingulate cortices and frontal eye fields have higher FDG uptake, while mesial temporal lobes typically have lower FDG uptake compared to other cortices.*

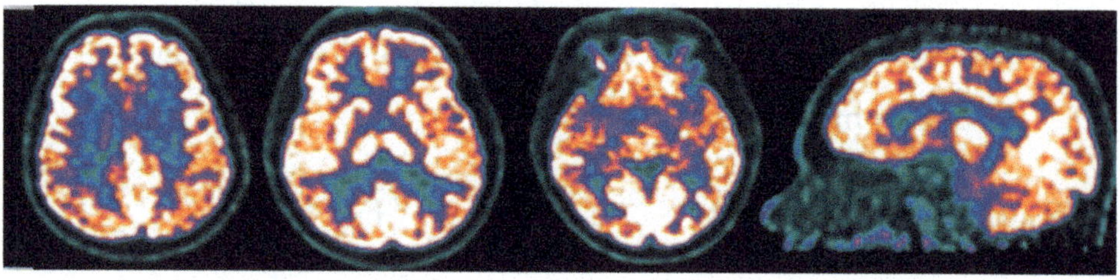

Dementia

(Stereotactic surface projection (SSP) images with decreasing level of metabolism: colour red >yellow >green > blue)

Alzheimer's Disease (AD)

- *Decreased metabolism is noted in the posterior cingulate gyrus, precuneus and posterior parieto-temporal cortices with preserved uptake in primary sensorimotor and occipital cortex. Frontal cortices can be involved in advanced cases.*

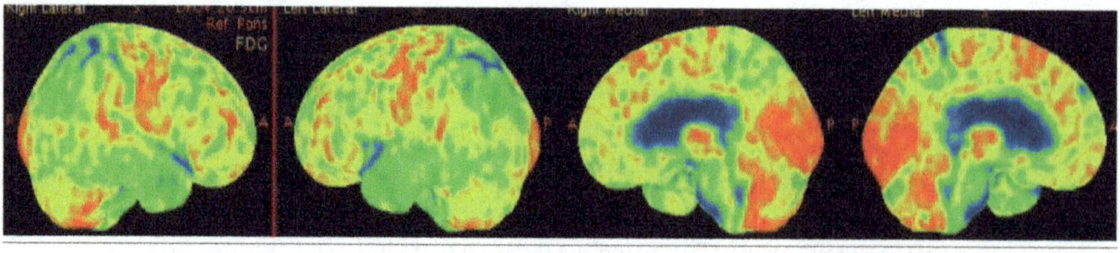

Fronto-Temporal Dementia (FTD)

Decreased metabolism is noted in anterior cingulate gyrus,and frontal or anterior temporal cortex (based on subtype).

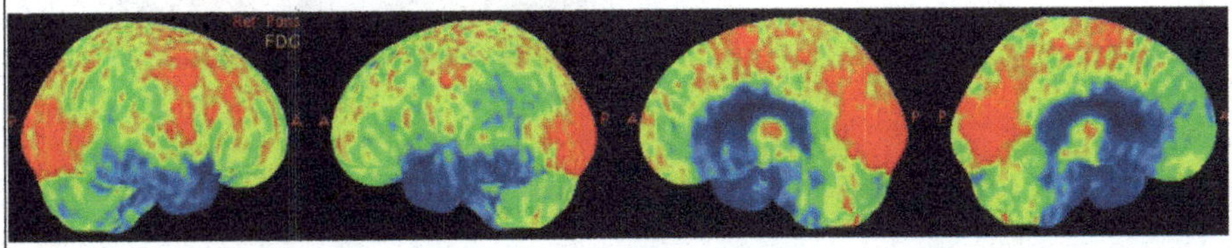

Corticobasal GanglionicDegeneration (CBGD)

Asymmetrically decreased uptake in bilateral cerebral cortices and basal ganglia.

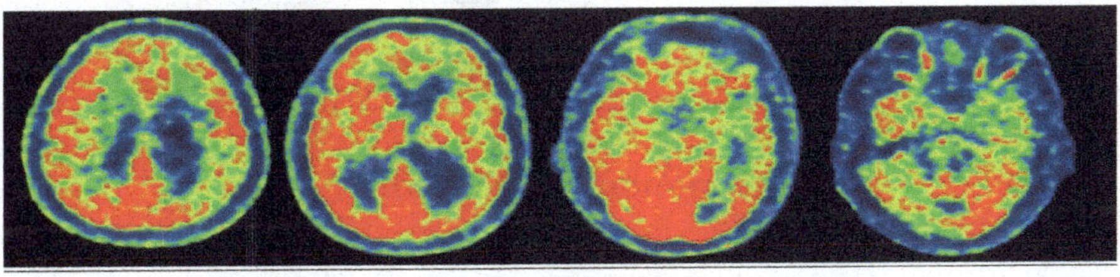

Atypical Parkinsonian Syndromes

- **Progressive supranuclear palsy (PSP):** *Decreased metabolism is seen in the medial frontal cortices, mid brain, caudate nucleus and thalamus*

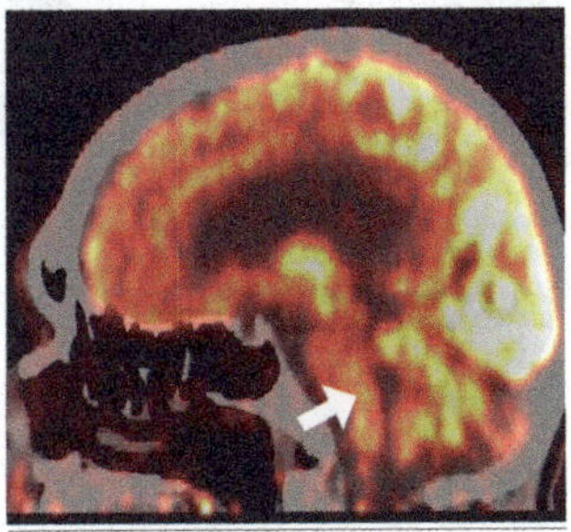

<table>
<tr><td>

• **Multi System Atrophy – Cerebellar type (MSA-C)**

Decreased metabolism is noted in the bilateral cerebellar hemispheres

</td><td colspan="2">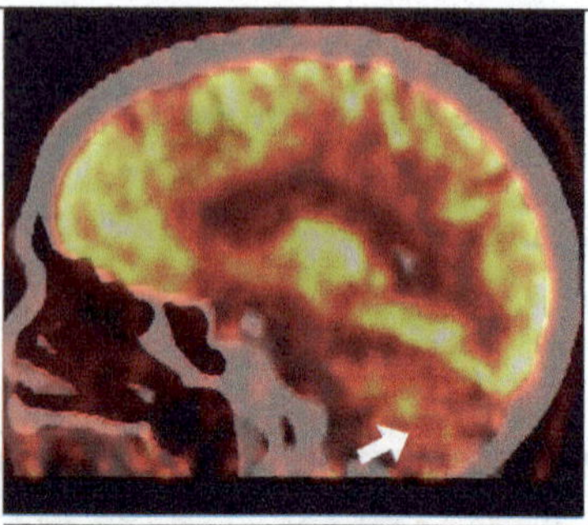</td></tr>
<tr><td colspan="3">

Localization of epileptogenic focus

</td></tr>
<tr><td>

• **Mesial temporal lobe epilepsy**

Decreased metabolism is noted in the epileptogenic focus in the right mesial temporal cortex.

</td><td colspan="2">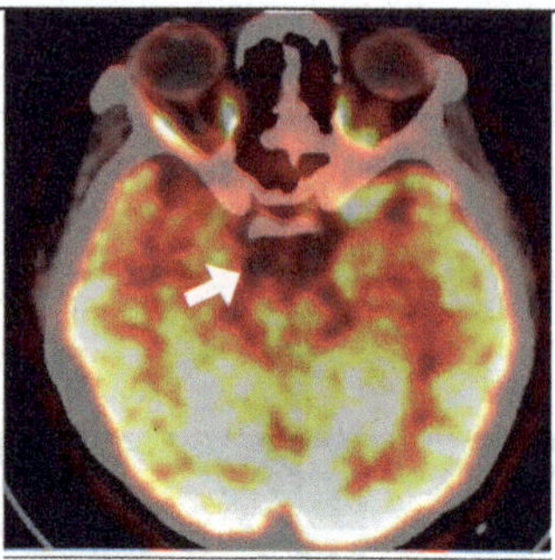</td></tr>
<tr><td colspan="3">

Autoimmune Encephalitis

</td></tr>
<tr><td>

- *Findings depend upon the receptors involved.*
- *Increased metabolism is typically noted in basal ganglia and mesial temporal cortices/hippocampus.*
- *Decreased metabolism is noted in posterior temporal-parietal and occipital cortices.*

</td><td>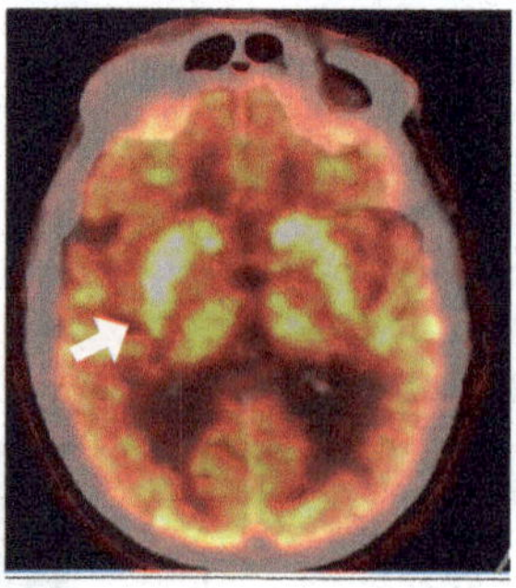</td><td>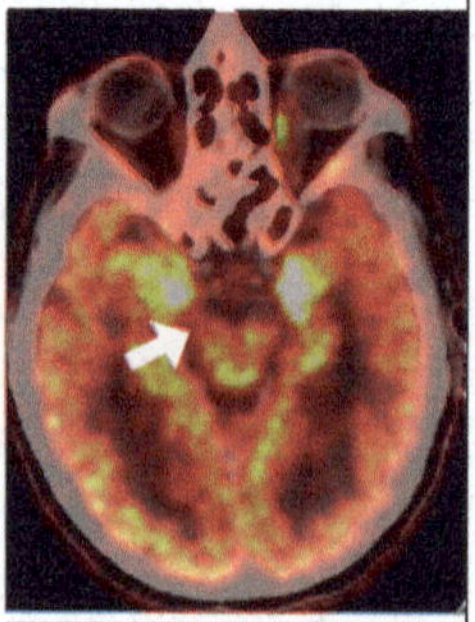</td></tr>
</table>

8.2 Dopaminergic System Imaging

Dopaminergic receptor imaging:

- ^{18}F – DOPA, a PET tracer, is a precursor for dopamine and enters the presynaptic dopaminergic neurons.
- ^{99m}Tc–TRODAT, a SPECT tracer, binds to the dopamine transporter (DAT) in the presynaptic dopaminergic neurons.
- Degeneration of dopaminergic neurons leads to reduced tracer uptake in the striatum in Parkinson's disease.

Radiopharmaceutical	^{18}F- DOPA	^{99m}Tc- TRODAT
Administration route	Intravenous	Intravenous
Dose (for adults)	4-5 mCi (148-185 MBq)	20 mCi (740 MBq)

Indications:

- For evaluation of idiopathic Parkinson's disease as the cause of movement disorders and differentiate from drug-induced Parkinsonism and essential tremors.
- ^{18}F-DOPA is also used for tumour imaging (neuroendocrine tumours; especially for insulinoma, medullary thyroid cancer, etc.)

^{18}F – DOPA PET/CT

Normal scan/Drug induced Parkinsonism/Essential tremors: *Both caudate nucleus and putamen show preserved tracer uptake.*

Early Parkinson's disease: *Asymmetrical decrease in tracer uptake noted in caudate nucleus and putamen (caudal putamen initially), contralateral to side of clinical signs.*

Late Parkinson's disease: *Symmetrical severe reduction in tracer uptake in caudate nucleus and putamen.*

Normal scan	Early Parkinson's disease	Late Parkinson's Disease
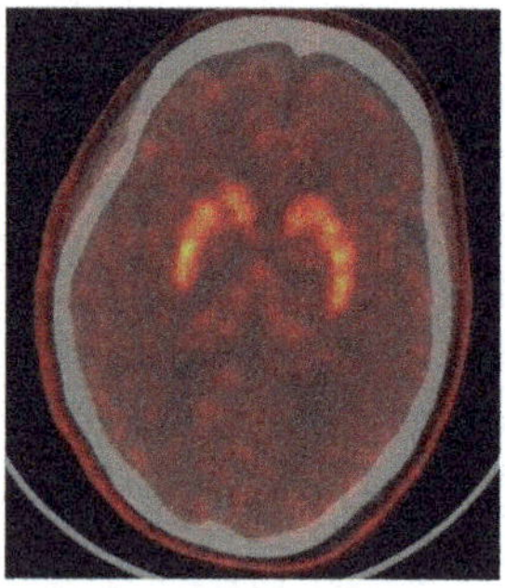	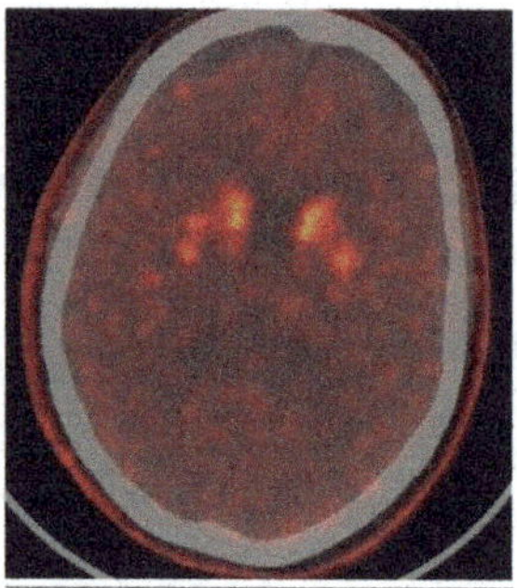	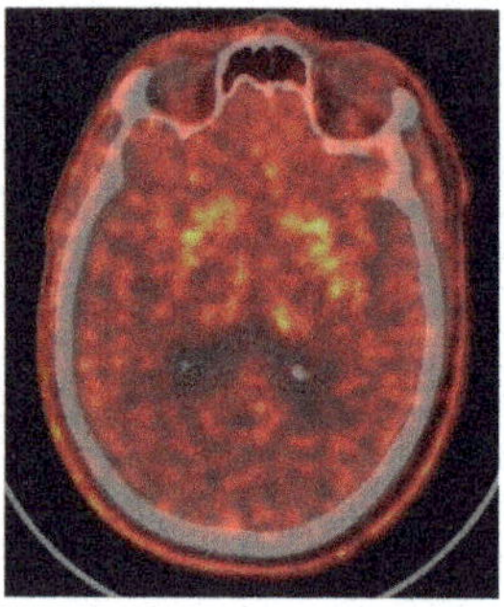

^{99m}Tc-TRODAT – SPECT

Similar biodistribution and findings as ^{18}F-DOPA PET but comparatively inferior image resolution. *A case of Parkinson's disease with predominantly left-sided tremors showing decreased uptake in right striatum.*	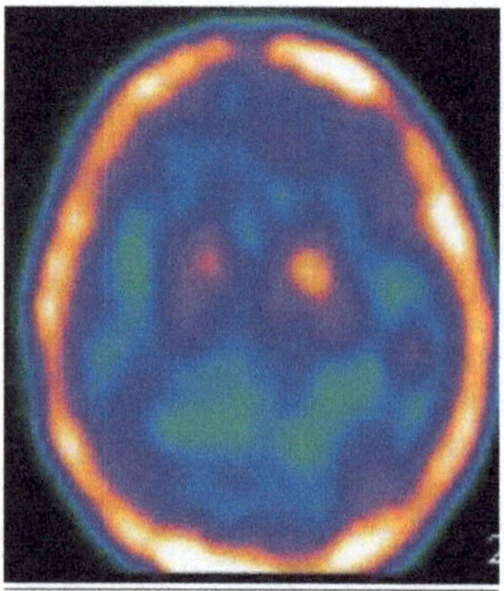

8.3 Brain Perfusion SPECT

^{99m}Tc based perfusion tracer SPECT imaging

- Lipophilic tracers such as ^{99m}Tc–hexamethylpropyleneamine oxime (HMPAO) and ^{99m}Tc-ethyl cysteinate dimer (ECD) are used, which penetrate the blood-brain barrier.
- Tracer uptake is proportional to the regional perfusion of the brain at the time of injection.

Radiopharmaceutical	**^{99m}Tc- HMPAO**	**^{99m}Tc- ECD**
Administration route	Intravenous	Intravenous
Dose (for adults)	15-20 mCi (555-740 MBq)	15-20 mCi (555-740 MBq)

Indications:

- For evaluation of regional cerebral perfusion defects – secondary to cerebrovascular disorders.
- For assessing perfusion improvement following vascular surgery.
- For assessment of dementias.
- For assessment of epileptogenic foci by Ictal SPECT and subtraction with Interictal SPECT.

Normal ^{99m}Tc – ECD brain perfusion SPECT/CT

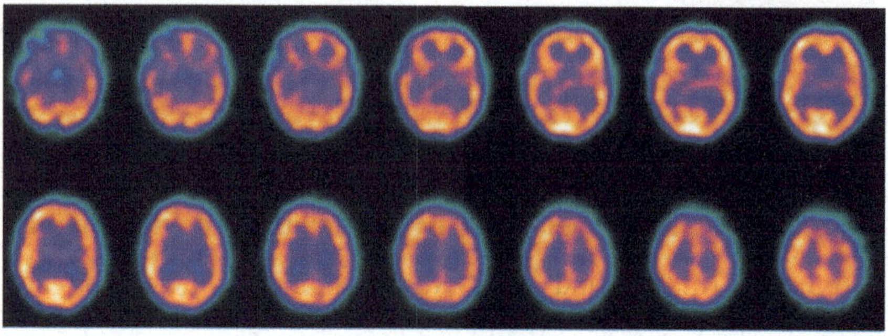

Symmetrical perfusion in bilateral cerebral cortices, cerebellum, basal ganglia and thalami.

Cerebrovascular disease

Region of reduced perfusion seen as a perfusion defect.

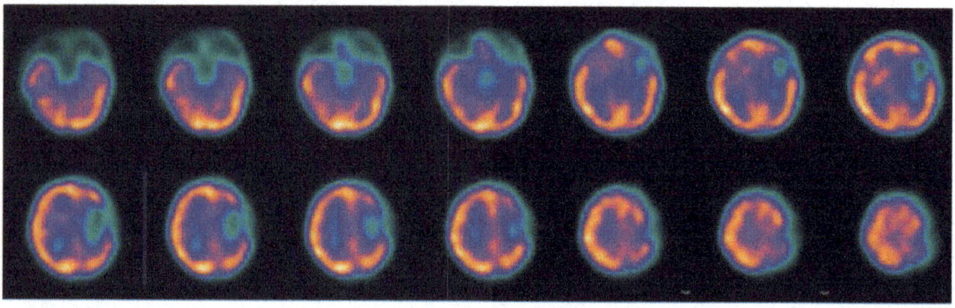

Perfusion defect is noted in left frontoparietal and anterior temporal cortices secondary to stroke.

8.4 Brain Tumour, Brain Death Imaging and Cisternography

1. Brain Tumour Imaging

Mechanism:

- SPECT tracers used are ^{99m}Tc – Glucoheptonate (GHA) and ^{99m}Tc – DTPA (also used as renal tracer). SPECT tracers localize tumours due to multiple factors like breakdown of the blood-brain barrier, increased vascularity, and permeability.
- PET tracers, which can be used, include ^{18}F-FDG and amino acid based tracers like ^{18}F-DOPA, ^{18}F-choline, ^{18}F-fluoroethyl-tyrosine (FET), etc. PET tracers localize based on the increased metabolism (FDG) or increased cell proliferation and amino acid utilization (DOPA, FET) of tumour cells, or other metabolic pathways.

Radiopharmaceutical	**^{99m}Tc – GHA SPECT**	**^{18}F – FDG PET**
Administration route	Intravenous	Intravenous
Dose (for adults)	20 mCi (740 MBq)	3-5 mCi (111-185 MBq)

Indications: The primary modality for evaluation of the brain tumours is MRI. Functional imaging is mainly used to distinguish post-treatment changes such as radiation necrosis from a residual tumour. It can also be used for radiation treatment planning.

2. Brain Death Imaging

Mechanism:

- ^{99m}Tc–DTPA is used for brain death scintigraphy.
- Following intravenous injection, blood flow in the cerebral cortices is seen on dynamic images in a normal patient.
- In a brain dead patient, the blood flow through the internal carotid circulation and to the brain is absent, and the tracer is diverted to the external carotid circulation.
- Findings include prominent visualization of nasal mucosa (‘*hot nose’ sign*) and the scalp, with non-visualization of brain parenchyma.

Indication: Assessing blood flow to the brain and identifying brain death when clinical and electroencephalographic findings are equivocal or inconclusive.

3. Cisternography

Mechanism:

- ^{99m}Tc–DTPA is used as an intrathecal injection. Tracer follows the normal pattern of cerebrospinal fluid (CSF) flow in the ventricular spaces, which is visualized by sequential static images. Any delay or non-visualization of CSF spaces is considered pathological.

Indication:

For assessing the presence of normal pressure hydrocephalus, CSF leak and patency of ventriculo-peritoneal shunt.

Section 9

Positron Emission Tomography (PET)

Dr. Swayamjeet S

Dr. Yamini Mathur

Dr. Rajender Kumar

9.1 ^{18}F-FDG PET-CT

2-[F-18]fluoro-2-deoxy-D-glucose (FDG)

- ^{18}F is a cyclotron-produced positron emitter with a half-life of 110 minutes, which can be used to label various pharmaceuticals (example, ^{18}F-FDG, ^{18}F-PSMA, ^{18}F-FET, etc.).
- ^{18}F-FDG is the most commonly used positron emission tomography (PET) radiopharmaceutical for a wide variety of oncological and non-oncological clinical indications.

Mechanism of uptake:

- ^{18}F-FDG is a glucose analogue with glucose transporter (GLUT) dependent uptake in metabolically active cells. It is trapped inside cells after phosphorylation by hexokinase, since it cannot be metabolized further and cannot diffuse out of the cell.
- The uptake of FDG varies for different tumour types. High number of viable tumour cells, high GLUT-1 expression, increased hexokinase activity and low glucose-6-phosphatase activity in tumour cells are associated with increased FDG uptake.
- ^{18}F-FDG is not a tumor specific agent and is used for imaging infection and inflammatory conditions as well.

Patient preparation:

	Recommendation	Rationale
Fasting	4-6 hours	To avoid insulin-dependent skeletal muscle uptake.
S. Glucose level	Should be <200 mg/dL.	To reduce competition with glucose/low insulin levels.
Good hydration	Before and after the injection.	To decrease FDG concentration in urine and radiation exposure.
Patient should be kept warm	30-60 minutes before tracer injection and 45-60 minutes after inj.	To avoid adrenergic stimulation and brown fat activation.
Insulin should be stopped	Short-acting - 4-6 hours. Intermediate-acting - 12-18 hours. Long-acting- 24 hours.	To avoid insulin-dependent skeletal muscle uptake.
Quiet and relaxed	Sit in a dimly lit room Shouldn't read, talk or be active	To avoid brain hyperactivity.
Void before scan	5 minutes before scan	High urinary bladder FDG concentration can impair pelvic lesion interpretation.
Breastfeeding	Stopped for 8-12 hours after injection	To avoid external radiation exposure to the infant.
Sedation	If patient cannot lie still for 15-20 minutes.	To avoid movement artefacts.

Special preparation:

- For cardiac sarcoidosis: Low carbohydrate and high-fat diet should be advised for at least 24 hours, followed by 12 hour overnight fasting before the scan.
- For myocardial viability assessment: see *section 6.3*

Clinical factors and recommended delay in ^{18}F-FDG PET/CT scan:

History	Recommendation	Rationale
Prior surgery	6-8 weeks delay (if the scan is required to assess for local recurrence).	False-positive due to inflammatory changes.
Chemotherapy	Delay for 3-4 weeks or plan before subsequent therapy.	To avoid false positive due to systemic effects.
Radiotherapy	Delay scan for 10-12 weeks.	False-positive due to radiation-induced inflammation.
Colony stimulating factors	Delay for 1-2 weeks.	Leads to bone marrow hypermetabolism.

Radiopharmaceutical	**^{18}F-FDG**
Route	Intravenous
Dose	7-10 mCi (260-370 MBq) for adults. 0.14-0.21 mCi (5.2-7.8 MBq)/kg for children.

mCi, Millicurie;MBq, Mega Becquerel.

Image acquisition: Images are acquired from skull base to mid-thigh, 45-60 minutes after injection. Brain and limbs may also be scanned, if required.

Clinical indications:

- **Oncological:**
  - Localization of primary tumour in cases of unknown primary.
  - **Staging**- when the tumour can be treated radically and baseline staging is required, e.g. Lymphoma, locally advanced ca. breast, ca. lung, etc.
  - **Response evaluation**- where further management depends on the response to therapy, e.g. lymphoma, multiple myeloma, etc.
  - **Recurrence or residual disease**: e.g. Brain tumors, head and neck cancer, ca. esophagus, ca. colon, ca. ovary, etc.
  - **Radiotherapy planning**: ca. lung, head and neck cancer, brain tumors, etc.
  - To localize primary tumor in **paraneoplastic syndromes**.

- Suspected **dedifferentiation** of tumor, e.g. neuroendocrine tumors, thyroid cancer, prostate cancer.
- Suspected **Richter's transformation** in low-grade lymphoma/leukemia.
- Differentiating radiation-induced necrosis from residual/recurrent brain tumour.
- PET-guided biopsy planning.

- **Non-oncological:**
  - Pyrexia of unknown origin (PUO).
  - **Brain:** Dementia, movement disorder and autoimmune encephalitis.
  - **Cardiac:** Myocardial viability, infective endocarditis, cardiac sarcoidosis.
  - **Lung:** Solitary pulmonary nodule assessment, infection.
  - **Skeletal system:** Prosthesis infection.
  - **Autoimmune diseases:** Large vessel vasculitis, Polymyalgia Rheumatica, IgG4 related disease, etc.

Quantitation in PET

Standardized uptake value (SUV) is the most widely used semi quantitative parameter in the PET-CT. It gives the relative concentration of the radiotracer (MBq/ml) in the ROI drawn on a lesion with respect to decay corrected injected dose (MBq) of radiopharmaceutical/unit body weight. SUV can be corrected for body weight (commonly used), lean body mass or body surface area. Maximum SUV within a ROI is called SUV_{max}.

Common pitfalls	
False Positive	**False Negative (Tumor with low FDG uptake)**
• Inflammation • Tumor hypoxia • Recent radiotherapy • Recent surgery • Recent chemotherapy • Hyperglycemia or hyperinsulinemia • Brown fat • Few benign neoplasms • Red bone marrow-anaemia, Granulocyte-Colony stimulating factor •	• Prostate cancer • Renal cell carcinoma • Hepatocellular carcinoma • Carcinoid • Mucinous adenocarcinoma • Low grade tumors • Differentiated thyroid cancer • Brain metastasis • MALT lymphoma • Well differentiated Neuroendocrine tumors (NET)

Common imaging patterns

Normal ^{18}F-FDG PET scan	***Physiological FDG uptake is seen in***
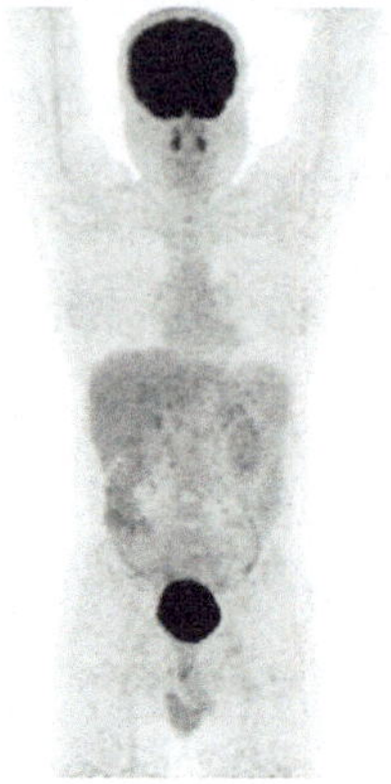 *Maximum intensity projection (MIP) image*	• *Brain (obligate glucose user)* • *Variable oropharyngeal activity (waldeyer's ring)* • *Moderate FDG uptake in the liver* • *Variable uptake in heart, GIT, salivary gland & testes* • *Kidney, ureter and urinary bladder (excretion)* • *Endometrial and ovarian uptake (related to the menstrual cycle)* • *Mild activity in bone marrow*

Brown fat uptake

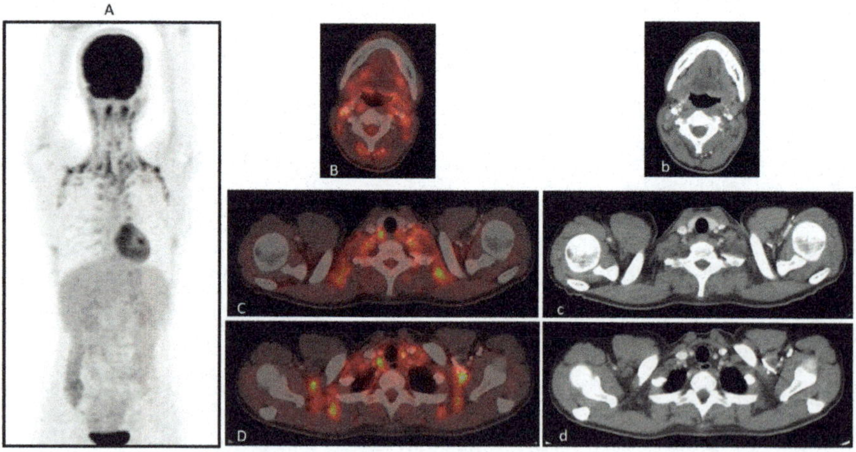

MIP image (A) showing physiological uptake in the brown adipose tissues in the bilateral cervical, supraclavicular, axillary and paraspinal regions (due to adrenergic stimulation). Axial cross-sectional hybrid PET/CT (B-D) and CT images (b-d).

Breast cancer

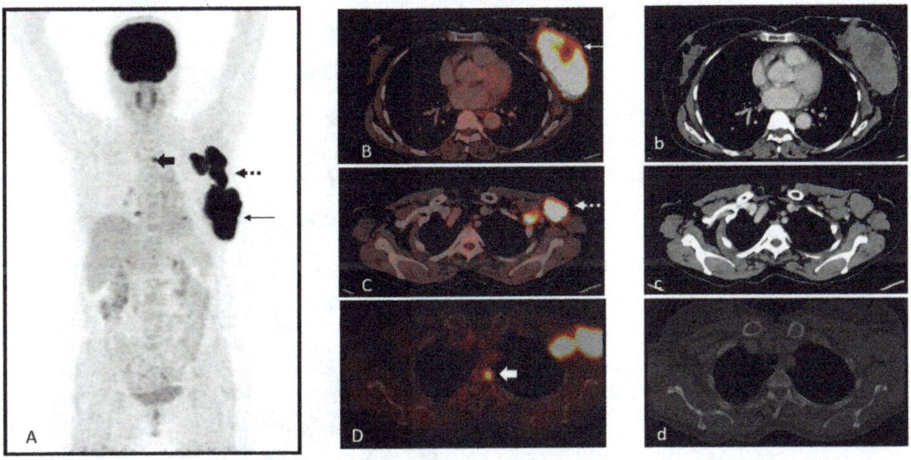

A 54 years old female patient of carcinoma left breast shows skeletal metastasis on staging ^{18}F-FDG PET/CT. MIP image (A) showing abnormal tracer uptake in the left chest region (line arrow), left axilla (dashed arrow) and in the midline of thoracic region (thick arrow). Hybrid PET/CT cross-sectional images showing FDG uptake in the primary breast mass (B, SUV_{max} 29.3), enlarged left level I-II axillary lymph nodes (C, SUV_{max} 22.9) and subtle sclerotic lesion in the D3 vertebra (D, SUV_{max} 9.1) suggestive of metastasis.

Hodgkin's lymphoma

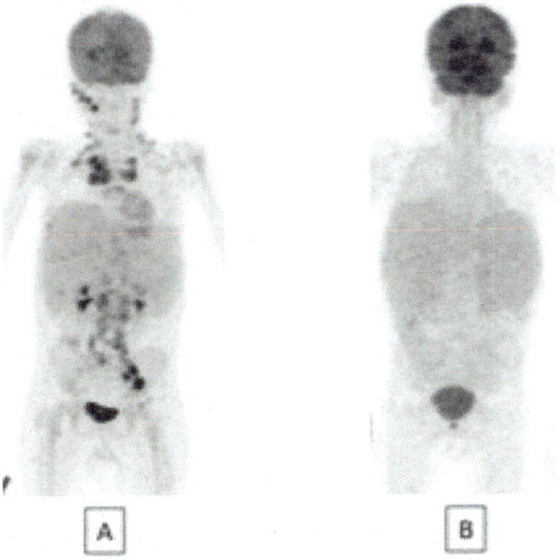

Staging PET scan of 9 years old child with Hodgkin's lymphoma (A), and interim response assessment scan post 3 cycles of chemotherapy (B). MIP image of staging PET scan (A) shows multiple metabolically active lesions (lymph nodes) above and below the diaphragm. MIP image of interim PET (B) showing complete metabolic response to therapy.

Vasculitis

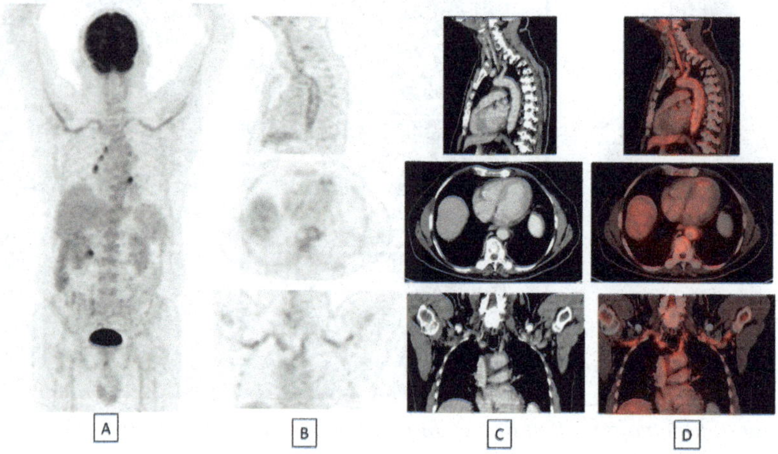

A 70 year old man with PUO for 7 months with a past history of treated Pott's spine (14 years back), was started on ATT again but showed no improvement. ^{18}*F-FDG PET MIP image (A) showing increased FDG uptake along the large blood vessels and foci of increased uptake in the thoracic region (mediastinal lymph nodes). Cross-sectional PET (B), CT (C) and hybrid PET/CT (D) images showing increased FDG uptake along the vessel wall thickening (descending thoracic aorta-* SUV_{max} *5.7) suggestive of active vasculitis.*

9.2 PSMA PET-CT

Mechanism:

- Prostate Specific Membrane Antigen (PSMA) is a 750 amino acid type II transmembrane glycoprotein.
- Shows increased expression in almost all prostate cancers; expression further increases in poorly differentiated, hormone-refractory and metastatic settings.
- Since the PSMA receptor allows endocytosis of the cell surface-bound proteins into an endosomal compartment, it can deliver the PSMA labelled radioisotopes inside the cell, thus making it an ideal theranostic agent.
- Currently, small molecule inhibitors of PSMA are used for imaging.

Radiopharmaceutical	**^{68}Ga-PSMA-11**	**^{18}F-PSMA-1007**
Route of administration	Intravenous	Intravenous
Dose	0.049-0.060 mCi/kg (1.8-2.2 MBq/kg)	0.1 mCi/kg (4 MBq/kg)
Excretion	Renal	Hepatobiliary

mCi, Millicurie;MBq, Mega Becquerel.

Indications:

- Staging of intermediate-to-high risk prostate cancer.
- Evaluation of biochemical recurrence after radical prostatectomy or pelvic radiotherapy.
- Restaging in non-metastatic castration-resistant prostate cancer (nmCRPC).
- Evaluation of disease extent in mCRPC.
- Planning for PSMA Radioligand therapy (see *section 11.4*).
- Assessment of response to systemic therapies.
- Planning for biopsy in patients with high clinical suspicion/prostate specific antigen (PSA) level after prior negative ultrasound or MR guided biopsy.

Patient Preparation:

- Fasting not required.
- Adequate hydration.

Scan protocol:

- Required activity (dose) of ^{68}Ga-PSMA-11 or ^{18}F-PSMA-1007 is injected intravenously.
- Scan acquisition begins 45-60 minutes later.
- Urine voiding required before scanning.
- Furosemide injection may additionally be considered shortly before or after ^{68}Ga-PSMA-11 injection to reduce urinary bladder activity.

Interpretation:

- Lesion with tracer uptake > surrounding background/blood pool is considered positive.
- Use of miPSMA (molecular imaging PSMA) score* improves specificity:
    - Score 0: uptake < blood pool
    - Score 1: uptake ≥ blood pool < liver
    - Score 2: uptake ≥ liver < parotid gland
    - Score 3: uptake ≥ parotid gland

Note: For ^{18}F-PSMA-1007, the spleen is the reference organ instead of liver. Scores 2 and 3 considered typical for prostate cancer lesions.

*Eiber M, Herrmann K, Calais J, et al. Prostate Cancer Molecular Imaging Standardized Evaluation (PROMISE): Proposed miTNM Classification for the Interpretation of PSMA-Ligand PET/CT. J Nucl Med 2018:59(3);469-478.

Imaging patterns	
^{68}Ga-PSMA-11 PET • *MIP image showing physiological distribution in salivary glands, lacrimal glands, kidneys, and bowel loops, liver, spleen, excretion into the urinary bladder.* • *Transaxial image showing PSMA expressing primary tumour in the prostate gland.*	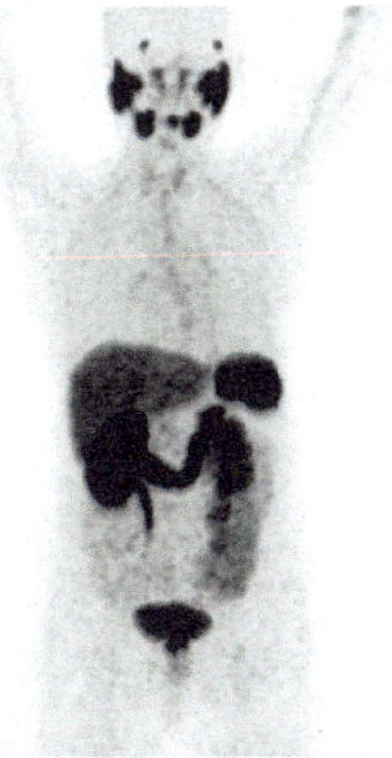 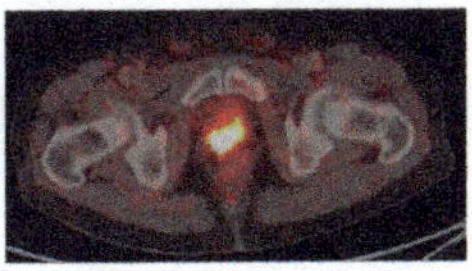

^{18}F-PSMA-1007 PET

- *Physiological distribution in salivary glands, lacrimal glands, kidneys, bowel loops, liver, and spleen.*
- *No urinary bladder activity (mainly Hepatobiliary excretion).*

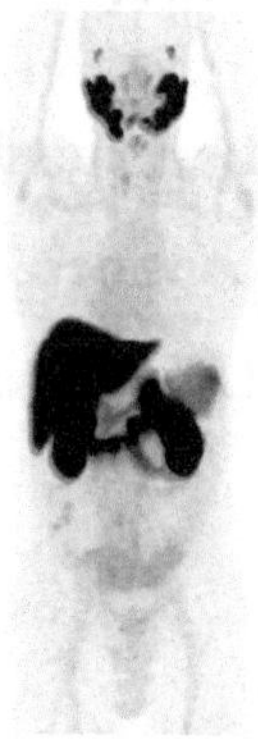

Staging of patient with high-risk prostate cancer (Gleason score 8, PSA 33 ng/mL).

- *^{68}Ga-PSMA PET showing tracer avid lesions in the prostate (primary) and multiple skeletal lesions (metastatic disease).*

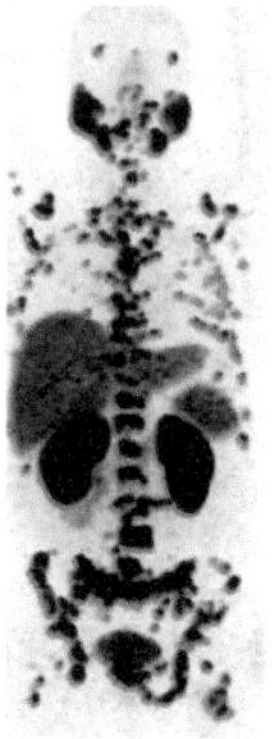

Response assessment after PSMA radioligand therapy

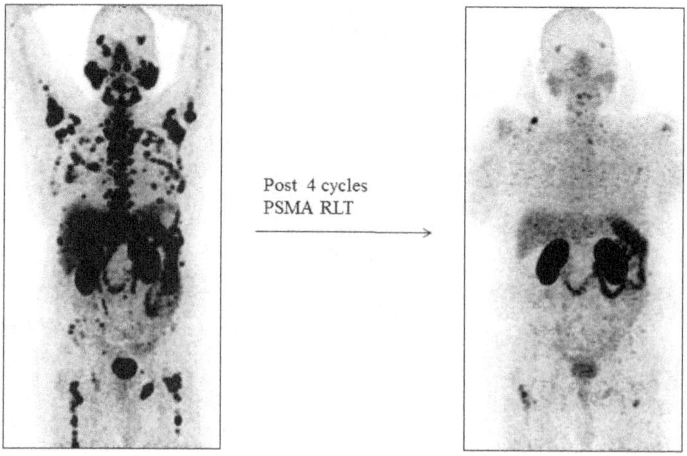

Baseline PSA 28.7 ng/mL

Post-therapy PSA 7.8 ng/mL

9.3 Somatostatin Receptor PET-CT

Mechanism:

- Target somatostatin receptors (SSTRs). SSTR-2 is most commonly overexpressed on neuroendocrine tumours (NETs).
- Radiolabelled somatostatin analogues (SSAs) are used for imaging and therapy.

Radiopharmaceutical	Abbreviation	SSTR subtype affinity
^{68}Ga-DOTA-Tyr^{3}-Octreotate	^{68}Ga-DOTATATE	2
^{68}Ga-DOTA-NaI^{3}-Octreotide	^{68}Ga-DOTANOC	2, 3, 5
^{68}Ga-DOTA-TyI^{3}-Octreotide	^{68}Ga-DOTATOC	2, 5

Indications:

- Neuroendocrine tumours:
    - Diagnosis and localisation of tumour in patients with high suspicion of NET.
    - Detection of unknown primary in a known case of metastatic NET.

- Staging of patients with histopathologically confirmed well-differentiated NETs.
- Response evaluation, restaging and recurrence evaluation.
- Planning for peptide receptor radionuclide therapy (PRRT, see *section 11.3*).

- Detection, staging, restaging and recurrence evaluation in Pheochromocytoma/Paraganglioma (especially extra-adrenal, SDH mutants, multifocal, or metastatic disease).
- Restaging and recurrence evaluation in Medullary Thyroid Carcinoma.
- Detection of neurogenic tumor in patients with suspected opsoclonus-myoclonus syndrome.
- Staging and restaging of patients with neuroblastoma.
- Detection of underlying phosphaturic mesenchymal tumors in cases of tumour-induced osteomalacia.

Note: *^{18}F-FDG PET/CT is useful for the evaluation of poorly differentiated NETs i.e. neuroendocrine carcinomas).*

Patient Preparation:

- Fasting is not required.
- Withdrawal of cold somatostatin analogues (3-4 weeks for long-acting; 24 hours for short-acting formulations) before the test.
- Adequate hydration.
- Breastfeeding: Interruption of 4 hours during which one meal should be discarded.

Scan protocol:

- 2.7-5.4 mCi (100-200 MBq) of the radiopharmaceutical is injected intravenously.
- Scan acquisition begins 45-60 minutes later.
- Voiding required before scanning.
- Three-phase CT may be acquired along with PET.

Common Imaging patterns	
Normal ^{68}Ga-DOTANOC PET scan *Physiological distribution in pituitary, spleen, adrenals, liver, kidneys; excretion into the urinary bladder. Variable uptake can be seen in the uncinate process of pancreas, salivary glands, thyroid, and bowel loops.*	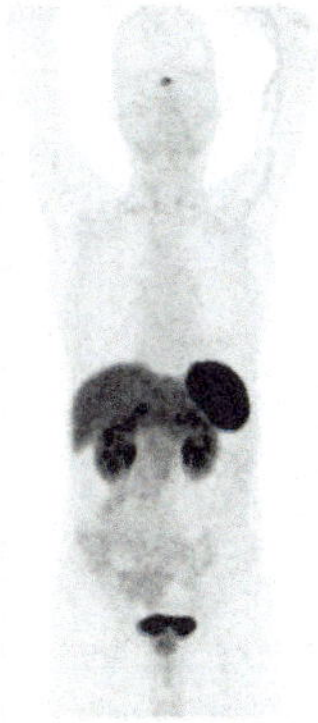
Staging of well-differentiated NET *SSTR expressing lesion in the pancreatic head– primary tumour.* *SSTR expressing abdominal lymph nodes and liver lesions– metastatic disease.*	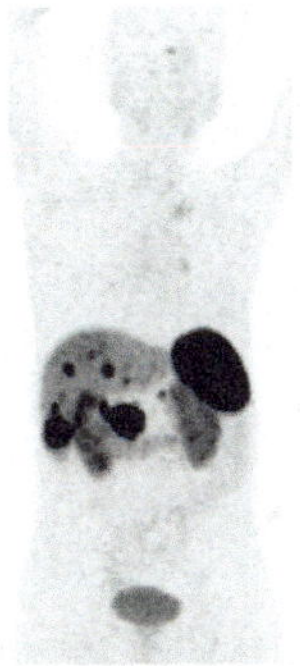 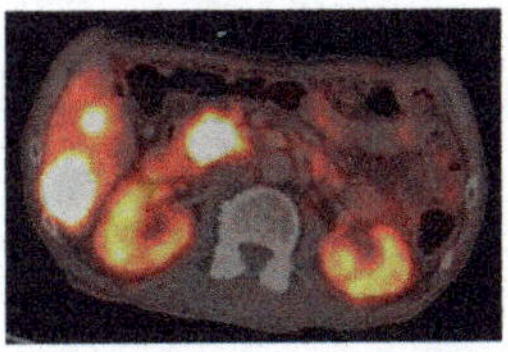

Paediatric patient with opsoclonus-myoclonus syndrome • *SSTR expressing left suprarenal lesion – Neuroblastoma.*	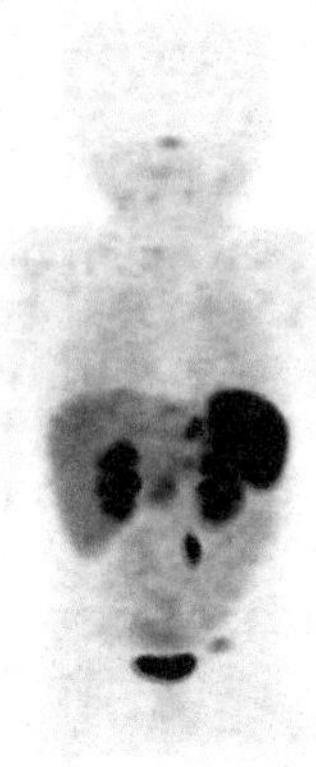

Section 10

Miscellaneous Investigations

Dr. TK Nitheesh Raj
Dr. Yamini Mathur
Dr. Karthikeyan
Dr. Harmandeep Singh
Prof. Anish Bhattacharya

10.1 Dacryoscintigraphy

Mechanism: The flow of tracer drop instilled into the eyes mimics the flow of tears.

Patient preparation: None.

Radiopharmaceutical	**^{99m}Tc – Pertechnetate**
Route of administration	Instillation of a drop of tracer on the conjunctiva.
Dose	0.05-0.1 mCi (1.8-3.7 MBq)

Indications:

- Diagnosis of tear flow/ lacrimal drainage disturbances.
- Follow up for detection of response to treatment.

Normal findings: The flow of tracer from conjunctiva to the nasal cavity via the nasolacrimal duct. Visualization of canaliculi within 10 seconds and the nasal activity within 10minutes. Normal findings exclude disturbances of tear flow with high probability.

Abnormal findings: Absent flow of tracer beyond the level of obstruction along the normal course of tears.

Advantages: High sensitivity and low radiation exposure.

Disadvantages: Low spatial resolution images.

10.2 Salivary Gland Scintigraphy

Mechanism: Salivary glands express the sodium iodide symporter, which takes up ^{99m}Tc-pertechnetate injected intravenously and excrete it into the saliva.

- Salivary gland scintigraphy is used to assess the functional status of the parotid and submandibular salivary glands.
- The functional status of sublingual glands and minor salivary glands cannot be assessed.

Patient preparation: No special preparation needed.

Radiopharmaceutical	**^{99m}Tc-Pertechnetate**
Route of administration	Intravenous
Dose (for adults)	8-10 mCi (296-370 MBq)

Indications:

To assesssalivary gland function:	Evaluate saliva secretion/duct patency:
Following irradiation	Following surgery (parotidectomy)
Sjogren's syndrome	Trauma
Salivary gland aplasia	Obstruction due to sialolithiasis

Imaging procedure: The patient is placed in the supine position and anterior images of the head region, including parotid and submandibular region are acquired for 30 minutes after intravenous injection of ^{99m}Tc-pertechnetate.

At 20 minutes of the acquisition (the time at which maximum salivary gland uptake of ^{99m}Tc-pertechnetate occurs), drops of lemon juice (as sialagogue) are instilled into the patient's mouth, and the patient is asked to swallow after 10 seconds. This is done to assess the drainage function of the salivary glands.

Common imaging patterns

Normal salivary scintigraphy: In a normally functioning salivary gland, the tracer uptake will gradually increase, and peak uptake occurs around 20 minutes after injection. After the instillation of lemon juice in an unobstructed gland, the drainage will be prompt, leading to a decrease in tracer activity in the salivary gland. The thyroid gland may be visualized.

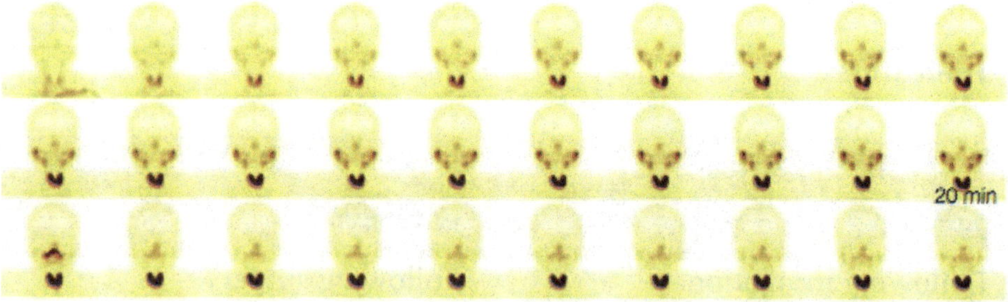

In the above images, the tracer uptake in both parotid and submandibular glands gradually increases, and peaks at 20 minutes.The drainage is prompt after the instillation of lemon juice at 20 minutes, indicating good salivary gland function and unobstructed drainage. Thyroid gland is also visualised in the neck.

Abnormal Salivary Scintigraphy:

- If the function of a salivary gland is impaired, the tracer uptake will be impaired, and the salivary gland will be faintly visualized.
- In an obstructed gland, after the instillation of lemon juice, the drainage will not be prompt, leading to the persistence of tracer activity in the affected salivary gland.
- In cases of severely impaired salivary gland function, drainage cannot be assessed due to negligible tracer uptake by the salivary glands.

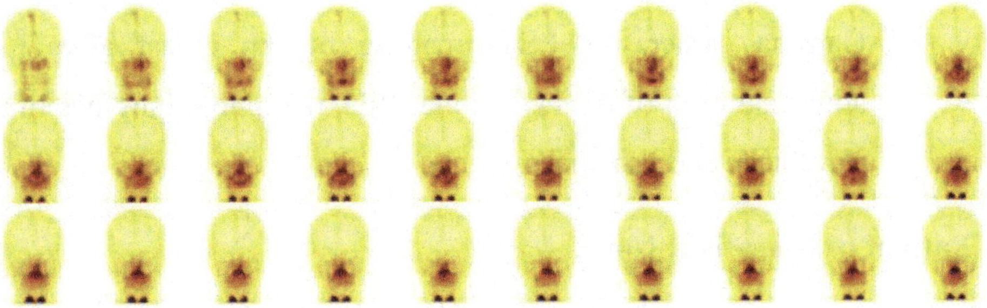

In the above images, there is negligible tracer uptake by the parotid and submandibular salivary glands, suggestive of severely impaired function, and drainage cannot be assessed.

10.3 Scintimammography

Mechanism:

- Use of tumour targeting radiotracers to detect suspected breast cancer. Tracer uptake is not dependent on increased vascularity or density of breast tissue, or mass formation. Thus, this can overcome the limitations of mammography.

- Gamma camera or PET imaging of the breast after i.v. administration of tracer is done. PET mammography has high resolution and sensitivity.

Patient preparation: None.

Radiopharmaceutical	**^{99m}Tc-Sestamibi**	**^{18}F-FDG PET**
Administration	Intravenous	Intravenous
Dose (for adults)	5-10 mCi (185-370 MBq)	2-3 mCi (74-111 MBq)

Indications:

- Breast cancer suspicion in high-risk women with dense breasts, breast implants, and for those who cannot undergo MR imaging.
- Adjunct to conventional breast imaging for problem solving in indeterminate cases.
- These modalities can also be used for evaluation for primary breast cancer in women with an unknown primary, to assess

extent of disease, evaluation of treatment response and detection of local recurrence.

Procedure:

- Static images of the breast in multiple planar views (Anterior, posterior, lateral) are acquired after radiotracer administration.
- PET imaging is done with ^{18}F-FDG.

Normal findings:

- Mild diffuse homogenous tracer uptake in bilateral breast parenchyma.

Abnormal findings:

- Focal increased tracer uptake with well delineated contours.
- Focal increased uptake in ipsilateral axilla (in the absence of any tracer extravasation) indicating lymph node involvement.

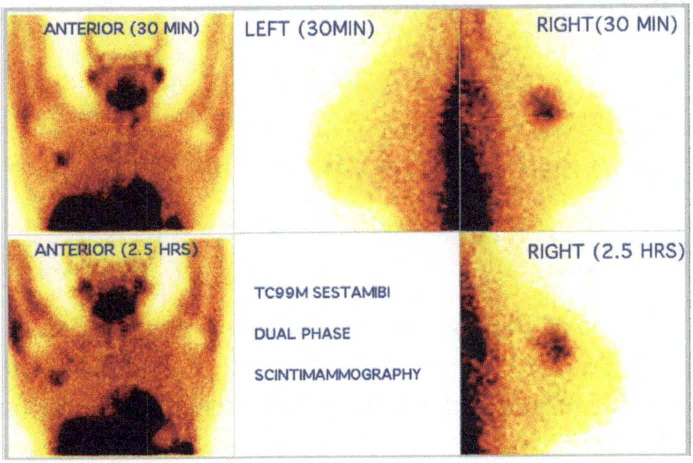

Scintimammography showing focal increased tracer uptake in right breast carcinoma.

10.4 Peritoneo-pleural Shunt Scintigraphy

Mechanism:

- Abnormal localization of a non-absorbable radiotracer to the thoracic region after administration into the abdomen/ peritoneal cavity.

Patient preparation: Presence of ascites is a prerequisite for the procedure. In the case of peritoneal dialysis (PD), no special preparation is needed.

Radiopharmaceutical	**^{99m}Tc – Sulphur Colloid or MAA particles**
Route of administration	Direct instillation of the tracer into the peritoneal cavity. Can use dialysis port in patients on PD.
Dose (for adults)	3-4 mCi (111-148 MBq)

Indications:

- Detection of the presence of Peritoneo-pleural leak or fistula in:
    - Patients with cirrhotic liver disease, liver or renal failure;
    - Patients on peritoneal dialysis: Peritoneo-pleural fistula is a rare complication of PD (1-5%). If present, PD needs to be discontinued.

Procedure:

- After confirming presence of ascites, instill tracer into the peritoneal cavity by direct injection.
- Agitate the patient's abdomen region.
- Acquire multiple static images of the abdomen (at 5 and 15 minutes after tracer instillation) and thorax (at 1, 2, 3, 4, 6 and 24 hours after tracer instillation).

Imaging patterns

Normal findings (No Peritoneo-pleural leak/fistula): The tracer is limited to the peritoneal cavity.

Abnormal findings (Peritoneo-pleural leak/fistula): Presence of tracer in the thoracic cavity (commonly on the right side). Delayed images at 24 hours are more useful in cases with minimal leak.

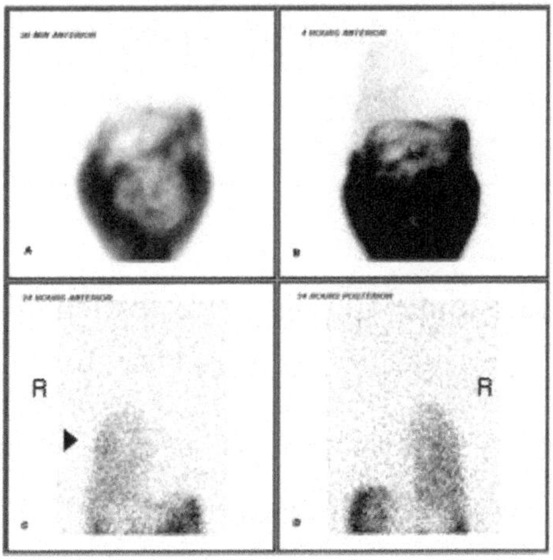

Serial anterior views of abdomen and thorax after intra-peritoneal instillation of the tracer. Initial 30-minute image shows tracer localisation in abdominal cavity with appearance of tracer activity in the right hemithorax on delayed images, suggestive of presence of peritoneo-pleural fistula.

10.5 Testicular Scintigraphy

Mechanism:

- Perfusion imaging to assess blood flow in testicular torsion.
- To evaluate regional abnormalities in blood flow and drainage.
- Blood supply to the testis is by the testicular artery while the scrotum is supplied by superficial and deep pudendal arteries.

Patient preparation: None.

Radiopharmaceutical	**^{99m}Tc – Pertechnetate**	**^{99m}Tc - DTPA**
Administration	Intravenous	Intravenous
Dose	2-3 mCi (74-111 MBq) for children. 10-15 mCi (370-555 MBq) for adults.	Same as ^{99m}Tc – Pertechnetate.

Indications:

- To differentiate among acute testicular torsion, appendicular torsion & epididymo-orchitis.
- Testicular scintigraphy is useful in intravaginal testicular torsion seen in children and adults. Surgical intervention within 6-12 hours of symptom onset can preserve normal perfusion and prevent irreversible spermatogenic dysfunction.

Procedure:

- Expose the scrotal region of the patient under the field of view of the gamma camera. Displace and tape the penis cranially over the lower abdomen. Separate both the hemiscrotum with any light and straight metallic object.
- After intravenous administration of tracer, immediate sequential dynamic perfusion images are acquired for 2 minutes, followed by multiple static images with marker image acquired at 2, 5, 10 and 15 minutes.

Normal testicular scintigraphy findings:

Symmetrical and homogeneous distribution of the tracer in bilateral hemiscrotum on static images. Flow in the testicular artery is poorly visualized.

Abnormal findings: Intravaginal testicular torsion

- **Early phase (<5-7hours):** Normal or mildly decreased perfusion on the affected side in dynamic images, with decreased tracer activity on static images.
- **Late phase (7-24hours):** Absent perfusion and hyperaemic ring secondary to inflammation with progressively increasing activity surrounding the affected testis (*Halo sign/ Rim sign/ Bull's eye sign*). Appendicular torsion can have variable appearance.

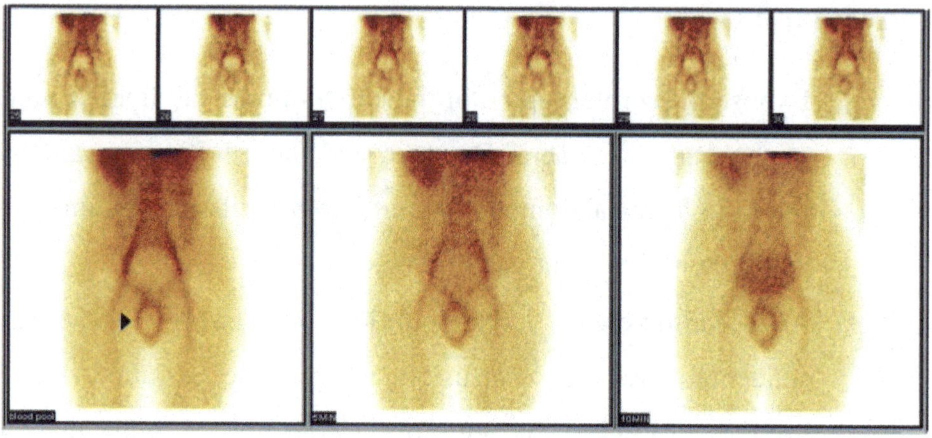

Blood flow, pool and 10 minutes images showing 'Halo sign' indicating late testicular torsion.

Conditions mimicking acute or missed torsion on testicular scintigraphy include abscess, hydrocele, hematoma and hernia.

Epididymo-orchitis: Increased perfusion and distribution of tracer on the affected side.

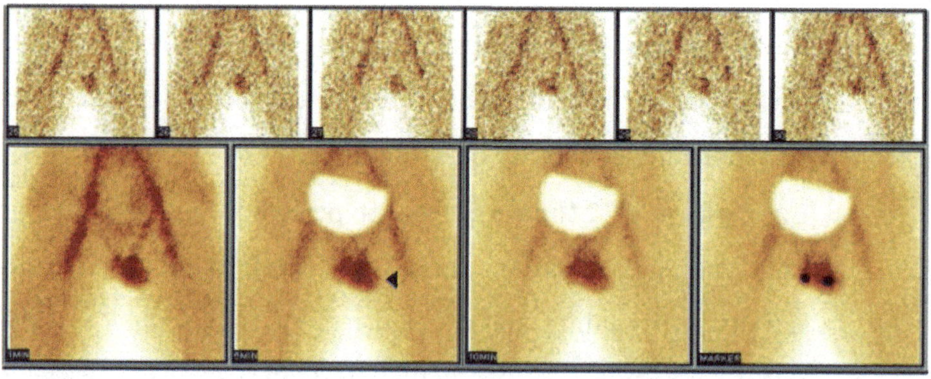

Blood flow, pool and 10 minutes images showing increased perfusion and tracer distribution in left hemiscrotum, indicating epididymo-orchitis.

10.6 Lymphoscintigraphy

Mechanism:

- Visualization of lymphatic drainage of particulate radiopharmaceuticals for the evaluation of lymphatic obstruction.
- One of the oldest practised nuclear medicine procedures.

Patient preparation:

The patient needs to wash hands/feet thoroughly before the procedure.

Contraindications:

Cellulitis/ gangrene at distal ends of extremities.

Radiopharmaceutical (^{99m}Tc – labelled particles)	**Particle size in nanometre (nm)**	**Dose (for adults)**
Antimony SC	<30 nm	1 mCi (37 MBq) in 1ml solution
Nanocolloid	<80 nm	
Sulphur colloid	100-600 nm	
Phytate	150-1000 nm	

mCi, Millicurie;MBq, Mega Becquerel.

Routes of administration:

- **Epifascial injection:**
  - Subcutaneous or intradermal injection in web spaces of feet/hands (commonly used).
- **Subfascial injection:**
  - Inject in the calf or along the lateral aspect of the foot at a depth of 1.5 cm (not done routinely).

Indications:

- To assess for lymphatic obstruction as cause of limb swelling.
  - *Differentials for limb swelling can be lymphedema, chronic venous insufficiency, deep venous thrombosis, lipedema, and other medical conditions (cardiac, renal or hepatic).*
- Prediction of lymphedema:
  - In contralateral limb in patients with unilateral lymphedema.
  - Secondary to surgery & radiation.
- Assessment of response to therapy.
- Localization of the site of leak in chylous ascites and chylothorax (with the help of SPECT/CT).

Procedure:

- Exercise of the extremities like walking for lower limbs, and handgrip exercise for upper limbs after injection increases the sensitivity.
- Images are acquired in both anterior and posterior projections at 10 minutes and 1 hour after tracer administration.

Normal Findings:

- Tracer activity is seen at injection sites in feet or hands.
- Near symmetrical visualization of tracer activity in inguinal or axillary lymph nodes by 1hour.
- Intercalary lymphnodes (popliteal or epitrochlear) are not visualized normally in epifascial injection but may be seen in subfascial injection technique.
- No backflow of lymph/tracer into dermal and subcutaneous lymphatics (*dermal backflow*).

Abnormal findings: Presence of any one of these findings suggests lymphatic obstruction:

- No movement of tracer from the injection site indicates complete lymphatic obstruction.
- The presence of dermal backflow indicates presence of lymphatic obstruction.
- Absent or asymmetrical visualization of inguinal (lower limb) or axillary (upper limb) lymph nodes on the affected side.
- Visualization of intercalary lymph nodes on the affected side.
- Extravasation or pooling of tracer.

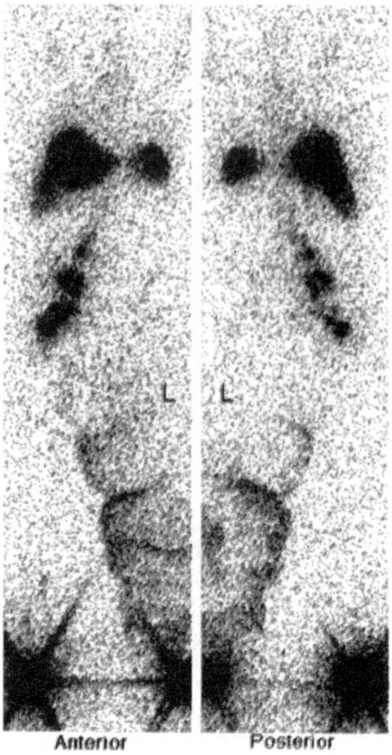

Lower limb Lymphoscintigraphy: Radiotracer activity is seen at injection sites in both feet. Normal lymphatic drainage is seen on the right side with good visualization of inguinal and iliac lymph nodes. Dermal backflow is seen on the left side (L) with non-visualization of inguinal lymph nodes, suggesting significant lymphatic obstruction. Liver activity is seen when lymph drains into the systemic circulation.

10.7 Intraoperative Gamma Probe

Intraoperative Gamma Probe

- Gamma probe is a hand-held device widely used in advanced centres for the ease and precision to guide surgery. The system has two components:
- **Detector system**- compact counting probe.
- **Electronic system** to amplify and process the signal to produce visual (in terms of count rate) and audio (in terms of frequency and intensity of sound) outputs.

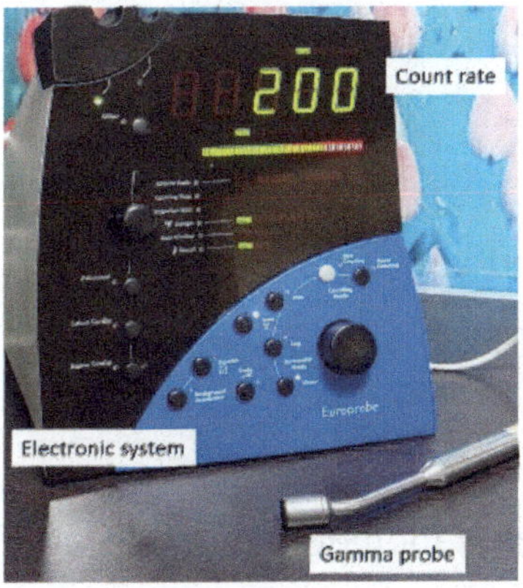

Intraoperative gamma probe

Applications:

A. Radio-guided sentinel lymph node biopsy (SLNB)
B. Radio-guided occult lesion localization (ROLL)
C. Radio-guided intraoperative margin evaluation (RIME)
D. Radio-immuno-guided surgery (RIGS)

A. RADIO-GUIDED SENTINEL LYMPH NODE BIOPSY:

- Sentinel lymph nodeis the first draining lymph node from the primary tumoral site.
- SLNB can be used as an indicator for lymph nodal metastasis in clinically N0 patients (e.g. no palpable node in breast cancer).
- Lymph nodal dissection can be avoided if tumour cells are absent in the SLN frozen section examination (in the same surgical setting), therefore, circumventing the long-term complications like lymphedema, limb pain, numbness, movement restriction etc.

Indications:

Most commonly used for early breast cancer and melanoma. Other tumours in which SLNB is employed are penile, vulvar, endometrial and cervical cancers.

Radiopharmaceuticals include radiocolloids (filtered/unfiltered ^{99m}Tc labeled sulphur colloid, Nano-colloids and antimony trisulfide) and Tilmanocept (LYMPHOSEEK).

Radiopharmaceuticals	^{99m}Tc labelled radiocolloids	^{99m}Tc labelled Tilmanocept (Lymphoseek)
Mechanism	Post phagocytosis lymph nodal fixation	Macrophage CD206 binding
Advantages	Readily available and cost effective	Stable, prolonged retention and rapid clearance from injection site
Disadvantages	Prolonged injection site retention and faster clearance from first echelon LNs.	Limited availability and expensive compared to radiocolloids

Patient preparation: No specific preparation is required.

Procedure:

- **Injection:** peritumoral or intra-tumoral intradermal/ subcutaneous injection is given. (In case of breast, peri-areolar intradermal injection is preferred.)
- **Imaging:** Planar and SPECT/CT imaging for lymph node mapping.
- **Skin marking:** Using gamma probe pre-operatively, the site with maximum count rate (other than inj. site) is marked with marker.
- **Intra-operative radio-guided SLNB** using gamma probe. Lymph nodes with raised count rates are dissected and sent for frozen section.

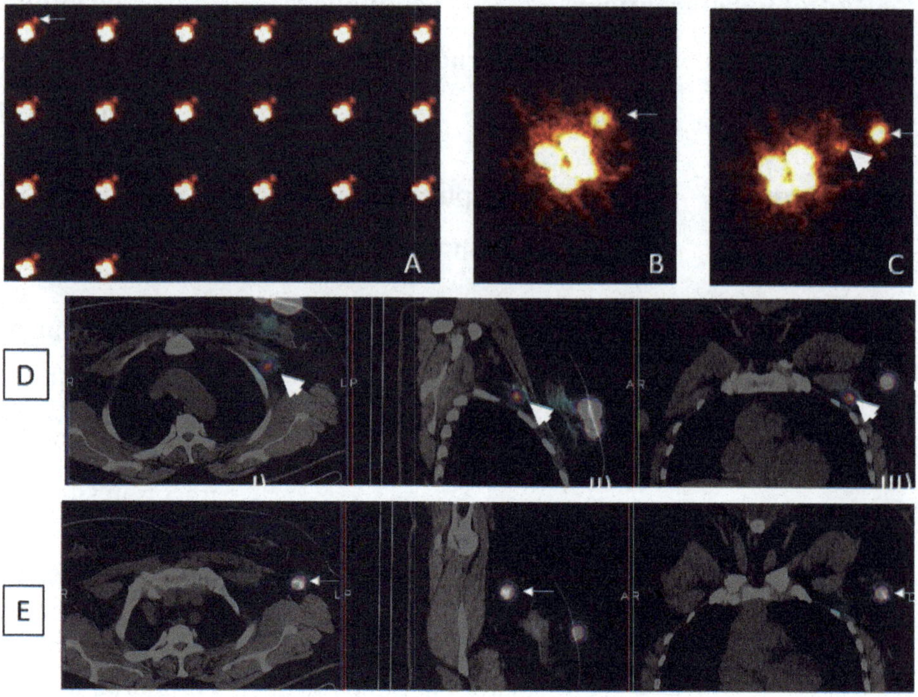

Sentinel lymph node mapping in a 54-year-old female with left breast cancer. Images acquired after peri-areolar, intradermal injections (4 sites) of 150-180μCi (5-7 MBq) of filtered ^{99m}Tc labelled sulphur colloid.

A. ***Dynamic image***: *Apart from intense injection site uptake, focus of increased uptake is seen in the left axillary region (arrow).*
B. ***Anterior planar image***: *Focus of increased uptake is seen in the left axillary region (arrow).*
C. ***Anterior left oblique planar image***: *showing an additional focus of tracer uptake (arrow head).*
D. ***SPECT/CT cross-sectional images*** *localizes the first focus to left level I axillary lymph node (Sentinel node) and second focus to left level II axillary node.*

B. Radio-guided occult lesion localization (ROLL):

ROLL is a minimally invasive procedure for intraoperative localization of a clinically occult lesion using gamma probe. It can be done by:

a. **Systemic administration** of a radioisotope labelled with a carrier, which has tropism for specific tumour or tissue. E.g., ^{99m}Tc-sestamibi for localization of parathyroid adenoma.

b. **Intra-tumoral administration** of a radiocolloid guided by imaging (CT/USG), e.g. USG guided intra-tumoral ^{99m}Tc-sulphur colloid administration in breast cancer.

C. **Radioguided intraoperative margin evaluation (RIME):**

RIME is an efficient technique, which uses intra-operative gamma probe to guide tumour resection and assess the adequacy of the surgical margins. E.g., intravenous 99mTc sestamibi in early carcinoma breast patient undergoing breast conservation surgery.

D. **Radio immuno guided surgery (RIGS):**

It is a new technique used for tumour detection using intraoperative gamma probe after intravenous injection of radiolabeled antibody. Most common investigated antibodies are:

- PSMA (Prostate Specific Membrane Antigen)
- CEA (Carcinoembryonic Antigen)
- TAG 72 (Tumour Associated Glycoprotein 72)

10.8 Infection and Inflammation Imaging

Mechanism:

Radiopharmaceuticals localize to the site of infection or inflammation by targeting different components of the inflammatory cascade.

Radiopharmaceutical	Mechanism of localization
^{18}F-FDG	Glucose metabolism in inflammatory cells at sites of inflammation.
Radiolabeled White blood cells (WBCs)*	WBCs localize to site of infection and inflammation by chemotaxis
^{67}Ga-citrate	Binds to lactoferrin and bacterial siderophores.

*Labelled with ^{99m}Tc HMPAO/^{111}In-oxine/^{18}F-FDG.

Other less commonly used radiopharmaceuticals include

- Radiolabeled monoclonal antibodies
- Radiolabeled chemotactic peptides
- ^{99m}Tc-ciprofloxacin
- ^{99m}Tc-Fanolesomab
- ^{99m}Tc-Sulesomab, etc.

In addition, 99mTc-MDP skeletal scintigraphy is useful for the diagnosis of osteomyelitis.

Imaging protocols:

Radiopharmaceutical	Patient preparation	Radiotracer Dose	Time of imaging
^{18}F-FDG PET	Fasting for 4 hours (see *section 9.1*).	7-10 mCi (260-370 MBq) for adults.	1 hour
Radiolabeled White blood cells (WBCs)	Patient's WBC count should be more than 5000 cells/mm^3. Invitro labelling facility needed.	^{111}In-oxine WBC 500 μCi (18.5 MBq) ^{99m}Tc HMPAO WBC 1-2 mCi (37-74 MBq)	24 hours 1-4 hours
^{67}Ga-citrate	No preparation needed.	5 mCi (185 MBq)	48 hours

μCi, microcurie; mCi, Millicurie;MBq, Mega Becquerel.

Indications:

- Pyrexia of unknown origin
- Osteomyelitis
  - Skull base osteomyelitis
  - Vertebral osteomyelitis
  - Diabetic foot
  - Infection at implant site/after trauma

- Lung
    - Infection
    - Inflammation: Sarcoidosis, pneumonitis.
- Cardiovascular system
    - Infection: Prosthesis/graft infection, endocarditis
    - Inflammation: Vasculitis
- Renal infection
- Abdominal infections and inflammatory conditions.

Section 11

Radionuclide Therapy

Dr. Sunil Kumar

Dr. Swayamjeet S

Dr. Jaya Shukla

Dr. Ashwani Sood

11.1 Radioactive Iodine Therapy for Hyperthyroidism

Thyrotoxicosis refers to the clinical syndrome of hypermetabolism when concentrations of free T4, T3 or both are very high. **Hyperthyroidism** refers to increased synthesis and release of thyroid hormone by the thyroid gland.

Radioactive Iodine therapy

- **Radioactive iodine (^{131}I) or RAI** is used to treat benign as well as malignant thyroid conditions.
- RAI therapy aims to treat hyperthyroidism by ablating sufficient thyroid tissue to achieve euthyroid or hypothyroid state.
- Sodium iodide symporter takes up ^{131}I, similar to natural iodine. The beta particles destroy the follicular cells, leading to volume reduction and control of thyrotoxicosis.

Radiopharmaceutical	Physical decay (Energy)	Half-life
^{131}I Sodium Iodide	β^- (0.606 MeV) γ (0.364MeV)	8.02 days

β^-, Beta; γ, Gamma

Indication:

- Hyperthyroidism due to Grave's disease, toxic adenoma and toxic MNG.
- Patients with recurrent thyrotoxicosis or having side effects of antithyroid drugs (ATD), cardiac arrhythmias, or thyrotoxic periodic paralysis.

Contraindications:

- Pregnancy, lactating mothers and children < 5 yrs. of age.
- Active thyroid ophthalmopathy& thyroid storm.
- Not able to comply with radiation safety precautions.

Eligibility criteria:

- Refractory or recurrent thyrotoxicosis after ATD therapy for at least 6 months.
- Recent thyroid function test (TFT) indicating hyperthyroid state.
- RAIU/^{99m}Tc-pertechnetate thyroid scan showing increased uptake of radiotracer in the thyroid gland.
- No active thyroid ophthalmopathy.
- No evidence of concomitant thyroid malignancy.

Treatment Protocol:

- ATDs should be stopped at least 5 days before therapy.
- No smoking (active or passive).
- 10-15 mCi (370-555 MBq) of ^{131}I-sodium iodide is given orally under supervision. A higher dose is given in patients with larger

gland and prolonged disease. Dose can also be calculated using RAIU value and thyroid volume.

- The patient is advised not to eat anything 2 hour before and after oral I-131 administration, and to take plenty of fluids for 1 week.
- Beta-blockers maybe administered for 6 weeks for palpitations, and analgesics in case of neck pain.
- ATDs if required, maybe started after 1 week for a short duration.
- **Radiation safety precautions**to be followed for one-week post-treatment.
- **Follow up after** 6 weeks with TFTs (TSH and free T4) and then every 3 months till the patient is euthyroid or stable on thyroid hormone replacement. Retreatment, if required, can be given after 6 months.

Therapeutic efficacy:

- 74% with 10 mCi and 81% with 15 mCi RAI therapy.
- TFTs normalize in most patients in 3-12 months.

Adverse effects:

- **Acute:** Metallic taste, dry mouth, pain and swelling in neck, thyroiditis, exacerbation of thyroid ophthalmopathy and transient hyperthyroidism (rare).
- **Late:** Hypothyroidism.

11.2 Radioactive Iodine Therapy for Thyroid Cancer

- Thyroid cancer constitutes 1-2% of all neoplasms and has a female preponderance.
- Four major types:
  - Papillary thyroid cancer (PTC) ~85%
  - Follicular thyroid cancer (FTC) ~10%
  - Medullary thyroid cancer ~3%
  - Anaplastic thyroid cancer ~1%
- Surgery is the mainstay of treatment.
- Postoperative radioactive iodine (RAI) treatment is useful.

Primary goals of postoperative RAI treatment:

- Remnant ablation –to facilitate detection of recurrent disease.
- Adjuvant therapy – decreases the risk of recurrence and disease-specific mortality by destroying suspected, but unproven metastatic disease.
- To treat known metastatic disease.

Radiopharmaceutical	Physical decay (Energy)	Half-life
^{131}I Sodium Iodide	β^- (0.606 MeV) γ (0.364 MeV)	8.02 days

β^-, Beta; γ, Gamma

Indications of RAI therapy:

- Primary tumour > 4cm or 1-4 cm with nodal metastases;
- Gross extra-thyroidal extension, extra-thyroidal or vascular invasion, aggressive histology;
- Iodine-avid pulmonary metastases;
- Unresectable iodine avid distant metastases;
- Recurrent iodine avid nodal and distant metastases.

Not recommended for unifocal tumour <1 cm with no high-risk features.

Eligibility criteria:

- Iodine avid disease on pre-therapy ^{131}I diagnostic whole body scan.
- No signs of marrow suppression (Hb, TLC and platelets within normal limits).
- No iodinated contrast study in the preceding 4-6 weeks.
- Willing to comply with radiation safety precautions.

Treatment protocol:

- Appropriate TSH levels **(>30mIU/L)** achieved either by thyroxine withdrawal for 3-4 weeks or after administration of recombinant human thyroid stimulating hormone (rhTSH).
- **Pre-therapy ^{131}I whole body scan** is performed 48 hours after oral administration of low dose I-131 (1.5 -2 mCi). SPECT/CT images can also be acquired to localise suspicious lesions.
- **Therapeutic dose of RAI:** 30-50 mCi (1.11-1.85 GBq) for remnant ablation, 100 mCi (3.7 GBq) for intermediate-risk

disease, 150mCi (5.55 GBq) for lung metastases and 200 mCi (7.4 GBq) for bone metastases.

- **Radiation safety precautions** to be followed for one week.
- Post-therapy scan is done after 5-7 days (additional lesions may be seen in 10-26% of patients).
- **Long-term treatment:** Suppressive doses of thyroxine and calcium supplementation are given.
- **Follow-up:** Patient followed every 6 months with **serum Thyroglobulin (Tg), Anti-Tg, TSH and calcium levels. USG neck** every 6 -12 months along with diagnostic WBS, if indicated.
    - Treatment can be repeated after 6 months for recurrent/residual iodine-avid disease till cumulative dose of approx.1Ci (37 GBq) is achieved;
    - Or till imaging is negative and stimulated Tg levels < 1 ng/ml.

Efficacy:

- **Low-risk patients:** 86-91% have excellent response (negative imaging and stimulated Tg levels < 1ng/ml).
- **Intermediate-risk patients:** 21-22% have biochemically incomplete response (negative imaging and stimulated Tg levels >10ng/ml);19-28% have structural incomplete response (structural or functional evidence of disease).
- **High-risk patients:** 67-75% have a structural incomplete response.

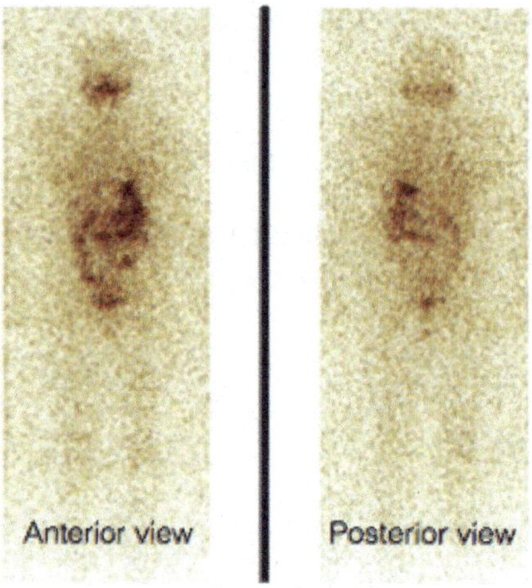

Negative Diagnostic ^{131}I-Scan, post thyroidectomy.

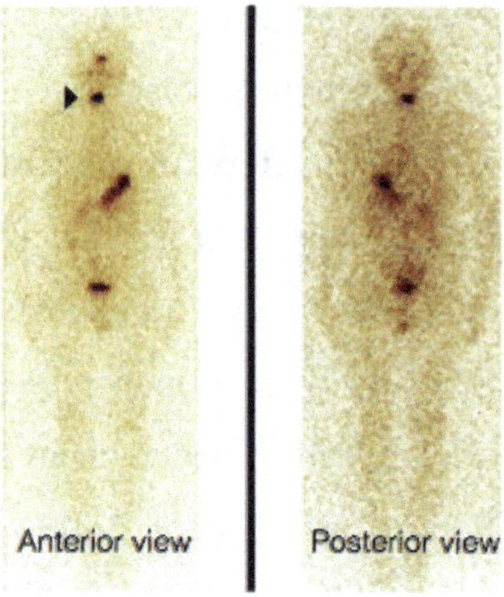

Tracer uptake in thyroid remnant on ^{131}I-whole body scan after thyroidectomy.

Adverse effects:

- **Early:** Nausea, vomiting, gastritis, radiation thyroiditis (in larger remnants), tumour swelling, bone marrow suppression (transient), xerostomia (all adverse effects are rare).
- **Late:** Radiation pulmonary fibrosis (<1%), secondary malignancies (leukaemia and solid tumours, <1%), bone marrow suppression, azospermia, and chronic sialadenitis.

11.3 Peptide Receptor Radionuclide Therapy (PRRT)

- Type of molecular targeted receptor-based radiopeptide therapy.
- Targets somatostatin receptors (SSTRs). SSTR 2 is most commonly overexpressed in neuroendocrine tumours (NETs).
- PRRT agents bind to the transmembrane SSTRs and are transported into the tumour cell by endocytosis, thereby causing DNA damage and cell killing.
- Currently, radiolabelled somatostatin analogues (SSAs) are used for PRRT.

Radiopharmaceuticals	**^{90}Y-PRRT**	**^{177}Lu-PRRT**	**^{225}Ac-PRRT**
Physical decay	β^-	β^-, γ	α
Half-life	64.2 hours	6.7 days	10 days
Agents	^{90}Y-DOTATOC	^{177}Lu-DOTATATE; ^{177}Lu-DOTATOC	^{225}Ac-DOTATATE; ^{225}Ac-DOTATOC

β^-, Beta; γ, Gamma; α, alpha.

- Currently, ^{177}Lu-DOTATATE is the only FDA-approved agent for SSTR positive gastroenteropancreatic NETs (GEP-NETs).

Indications:

- Advanced, inoperable/metastatic, progressive well-differentiated NETs.
- Inoperable/ metastatic medullary thyroid carcinoma.
- Non ^{131}I-MIBG avid metastatic pheochromocytoma and paraganglioma.
- Stage III/IV neuroblastoma, metastatic merkel cell carcinoma, and meningioma.

Eligibility Criteria:

- Lesions should have *high-grade uptake (> physiological liver uptake)* on SSTR PET/CT (^{68}Ga-DOTATATE or ^{68}Ga-DOTANOC PET/CT) or SSTR scintigraphy (^{99m}Tc-HYNIC-TOC SPECT/CT);
- No discordant FDG positive, SSTR negative lesion(s);
- Preserved renal function (eGFR $\geq$ 50 mL/min, creatinine <1.7mg/dL);
- Stable haematological parameters: Haemoglobin $\geq$ 8 g/dL, leucocytes $\geq$ 2000/µL, and platelets $\geq$ 70000/µL;
- Adequate liver function: Bilirubin < 3.0 x upper limit of normal (ULN); Albumin $\geq$ 3.0 g/dL.

Treatment Protocol:

- Long-acting SSAs need to be discontinued for 4 weeks before PRRT. They may be started 24 hours after PRRT. For symptomatic patients and poorly controlled functional NETs, short-acting subcutaneous SSAs can be given till one day before PRRT.

- ^{177}Lu-DOTATATE: 200 mCi (7.4 GBq) per cycle and ^{225}Ac-DOTATATE: 2.7 μCi/kg (100 kBq/kg) per cycle; slow IV over 30 minutes.
- Adequate hydration and nephroprotection comprising positively amino acids lysine and arginine (25gm each in 2 litre normal saline infused over 4 hrs, starting 30–60 min before PRRT).
- Prophylactic anti-emetics: i.v. Ondansetron, Dexamethasone.
- Time interval between cycles: 8-12 weeks.
- Number of cycles: 4-5 (depending on the response, prognosis, and renal status).
- Concomitant chemotherapy:
    - SSTR +ve and FDG +ve tumours (usually Ki 67 10-20% or 20-30%): 2 cycles of CAPTEM between 2 PRRT cycles;
    - Radiosensitizing role of low-dose Capecitabine (1250 mg/m^2 on days 0-14 of each PRRT cycle).
- Follow-up:
    - Every 3 weeks with CBC, LFT, RFT;
    - ^{68}Ga-SSA PET/CT and serum Chromogranin A at 6-8 weeks after 2nd cycle and 4th cycle.

Therapeutic efficacy:

Objective radiological response rate: 30-40%.

NETTER 1 trial*	^{177}Lu-DOTATATE + 30 mg Octreotide LAR	Octreotide LAR 60 mg
Objective RR	18%	3%
PFS rate at 20 months	65.2%	10.8%

*RR, Radiological response. *Strosberg J, El-Haddad G, Wolin E, et al. Phase 3 Trial of ^{177}Lu-Dotatate for Midgut Neuroendocrine Tumors. N Engl J Med. 2017 12;376(2):125-135.*

Toxicity:

- **Acute/early:** Nausea, vomiting, carcinoid crisis, myelosuppression, and nephrotoxicity.
- **Late:** Myelodysplastic syndrome, acute myeloid leukaemia (rare, <2%).

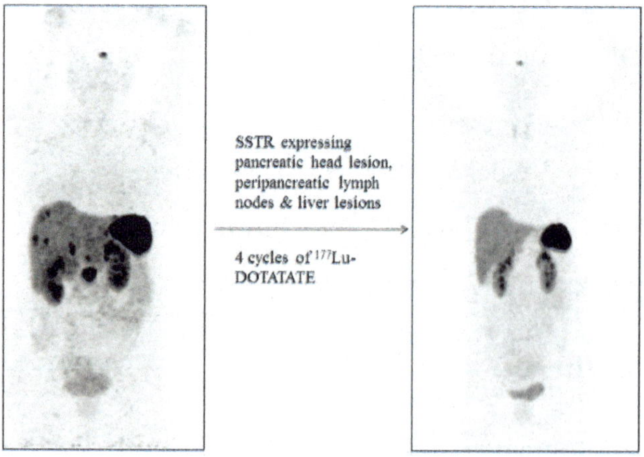

68Ga-DOTANOC PET-CT before and after PRRT showing good treatment response.

11.4 PSMA Radioligand Therapy

Prostate Specific Membrane Antigen (PSMA)

- 750 amino acid type II transmembrane glycoprotein.
- Increased expression in almost all prostate cancers; expression further increases in poorly differentiated, hormone-refractory, and metastatic settings. Since the PSMA receptor allows endocytosis of the cell surface-bound proteins into an endosomal compartment, it can deliver the PSMA labelled radioisotopes inside the cell, making it an ideal theranostic agent.
- Currently, small molecule inhibitors of PSMA are used for Radioligand Therapy (RLT).

Radiopharmaceuticals	^{177}Lu-PSMA-RLT	^{225}Ac-PSMA-RLT
Physical decay	β^-, γ	α
Half life	6.7 days	10 days
Agents	^{177}Lu-PSMA-617; ^{177}Lu-PSMA-I&T	^{225}Ac-PSMA-617; ^{225}Ac-PSMA-I&T

β^-, Beta; γ, Gamma; α, alpha.

Current Role:

- Currently reserved as salvage/compassionate treatment option.

- For patients with end-stage metastatic castration-resistant prostate cancer (mCRPC) who have failed existing treatment modalities.
- Increasingly being tried as upfront frontline therapy with favourable outcomes.

Eligibility Criteria:

- Biopsy-proven adenocarcinoma prostate;
- Metastatic disease (as established by ^{68}Ga-PSMA PET/CT);
- Significant PSMA expression in ^{68}Ga-PSMA PET/CT defined as lesion uptake being significantly (1.5 x) higher than normal liver uptake;
- GFR ≥ 30 mL/min;
- Stable haematological parameters: Haemoglobin ≥ 8 g/dL; neutrophils ≥ 1500/μL, and platelets ≥ 70000/μL;
- Adequate liver function: Bilirubin < 1.5 x upper limit of normal (ULN); AST or ALT ≤ 1.5 x ULN (or ≤ 5.0 x ULN in the presence of liver metastases); Albumin ≥ 2.5 g/dL;
- ECOG performance 0-2.

Treatment Protocol:

- 160-230 mCi (6.0-8.5 GBq)per cycle of ^{177}Lu-PSMA-RLT;
- 2.7 μCi/kg (100 kBq/kg) per cycle of ^{225}Ac-PSMA-RLT; slow IV with adequate hydration;
- Prophylactic anti-emetics: Ondansetron, Dexamethasone.
- Time interval between cycles: 6–8 weeks;
- Number of cycles: 2-6 (depending on the response, prognosis, and renal risk factors);

- No radiotherapy or chemotherapy within 4 weeks; continue ADT;
- Follow-up:
  - Every 3 weeks with complete blood counts, liver and renal function tests, PSA;
  - ^{68}Ga-PSMA PET/CT after 6-8 weeks (after 2nd cycle and 4th cycle).

Therapeutic efficacy:

- ^{177}Lu-PSMA-RLT: Best PSA decline of ≥50% in 40-60% patients.

TheraP trial*	^{177}Lu-PSMA-617	Cabazitaxel
Best PSA response rate	66%	37%
PFS rate at 12 months	19%	3%

*Hofman MS, Emmett L, Sandhu S, et al. [177Lu]Lu-PSMA-617 versus cabazitaxel in patients with metastatic castration-resistant prostate cancer (TheraP): a randomised, open-label, phase 2 trial. Lancet. 2021;397(10276):797-804.

- ^{225}Ac-PSMA-RLT: Best PSA response rate is 50-75%.

Toxicity:

- Salivary and lacrimal glands are the organs at risk.
- Xerostomia, xerophthalmia, fatigue, bone pain flare and myelosuppression.

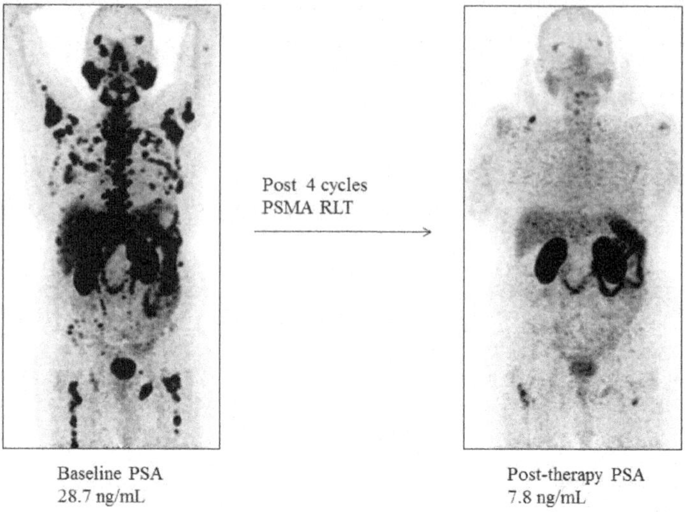

68Ga-PSMA PET-CT before and after PSMA RLT shows significant reduction in PSMA avid lesions, suggestive of significant response to treatment.

11.5 Metastatic Bone Pain Palliation Therapy

- Bone pain is a common presentation of skeletal metastases and is experienced to varying degrees by 60–90% of patients with advanced metastatic cancers.
- Metastatic bone pain can be treated with analgesics, bisphosphonates, hormonal therapy, chemotherapy, radiotherapy andradionuclide bone pain palliation therapy, alone or in combination.
- The radiopharmaceutical is adsorbed onto metastatic skeletal sites with increased osteoblastic activity. Alpha or beta emissions from the radionuclides lead to death of tumour and inflammatory cells and subsequent reduction of cytokines, growth factors, and periosteal swelling.
- Advantages of bone palliation radionuclide therapy:
  - Simultaneous treatment of multiple sites with a probable therapeutic effect on metastatic disease.
  - Ease of administration and retreatment.
  - Low toxicity and can be combined with other treatment options.

Indications:

- Refractory bone pain due to osteoblastic metastases from prostate, breast carcinomas, or other malignancies.

Contraindications:

- Pregnancy and lactation, metastatic superscan pattern on bone scan (due to extensive skeletal metastases with high risk of significant myelosuppression), and life expectancy < 3 months.

Radiopharmaceutical	Physical decay	Half life	Dose
$^{89}SrCl_2$	β^-	50.5 days	4 mCi (148 MBq) 40µCi/Kg (1.48 MBq/Kg)
^{153}Sm-EDTMP	β^-	1.93 days	1 mCi/Kg (37 MBq/Kg)
^{186}Re- HEDP **^{188}Re-HEDP**	β^-, γ	3.7 days 0.7 days	35 mCi (1.29 GBq)
^{177}Lu-EDTMP/DOTMP	β^-, γ	6.7 days	50 mCi (1.85 GBq)
^{223}RaCl2	α	11.4 days	1.35 µCi/Kg (50 KBq/Kg)

*$^{89}SrCl_2$ – Strontium-89 Chloride; ^{153}Sm-EDTMP – Samarium-153 ethylene diamine tetramethylene phosphonic acid; ^{186}Re- HEDP – Rhenium-186 hydroxyethylidine diphosphonate; ^{177}Lu-DOTMP–Lutetium-177 1,4,7,10-tetraazacyclododecane-1,4,7,10-tetramethylene phosphonic acid; ^{223}RaCl2 – Radium-223 chloride; µCi –micro curie; mCi-millicurie. MBq-Mega Becquerel; GBq-Giga Becquerel; KBq-Kilo Becquerel; β^-, Beta; γ, Gamma; α, alpha.

Eligibility criteria:

- Hb > 9gm/dl;
- TLC >3500/mm^3;
- Platelets >10^5/ mm^3;
- GFR > 30ml/min;
- ^{99m}Tc-MDP bone scan within 4 weeks showing increased tracer uptake at metastatic sites.

Treatment Protocol:

- Recent haematological and biochemical investigations (within 1 week).
- Painful metastatic sites on physical examination should correlate with the sites of increased radiotracer uptake on bone scan.
- Informed written consent from the patient.
- The radiopharmaceutical is administered by slow IV infusion followed by flush with normal saline.
- Radiation safety precautions for 1 week post-treatment.

Follow-up:

- Haematological investigations at 2, 4, 8and 12 weeks post-therapy.

Therapeutic efficacy:

- 60-80% of patients benefit from therapy. Pain reduction is seen at 2-4 weeks, and effects last for around 3-6 months.

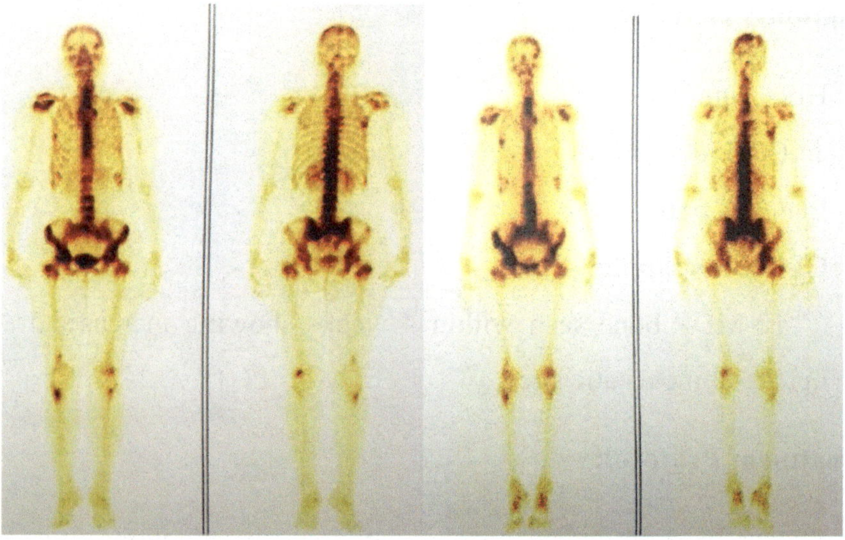

Pre-therapy ^{99m}Tc-MDP bone scan showing increased tracer uptake at multiple skeletal sites.

^{177}Lu-DOTMP post-therapy scan showing tracer uptake in skeletal metastases corresponding to bone scan.

Adverse effects:

- Pain flare in initial 1-2 weeks in about 10% of cases.
- Myelosuppression (transient decreased thrombocytes and leucocyte counts).

11.6 Selective Intra-arterial Radionuclide Therapy (SIRT)

Also known

as Trans-arterial radioembolization (TARE).

- Loco-regional therapy for liver cancer.
- Hepatocellular carcinoma (HCC) is the most common primary neoplasm of the liver.
- It is the sixth most commonly diagnosed cancer and the third leading cause of cancer deaths worldwide.
- Aetiology for HCC includes hepatitis, viral infections, alcohol, haemochromatosis, non-alcoholic steatohepatitis and diabetes.
- Liver-dominant metastatic site from neuroendocrine, bladder and colorectal cancers can also be treated with SIRT.
- SIRT targets to deliver 100-150 Gy radiation dose to the tumour.
- The unique feature of dual blood supply to liver is exploited to deliver radionuclide to tumour vasculature via hepatic artery, sparing the normal parenchyma.
- The commonly used radionuclides are Yttrium-90, Iodine-131 and Rhenium-188.
- Radiolabeled particulate formulations are preferred over radiolabeled lipiodol.

- Technetium-99m MAA scan plays an important role in pre-therapy dosimetry (shunt study).
- Triple phase CT and ^{18}F-FDG are useful in a) detection of distant metastases for therapy planning and b) SIRT response evaluation.

Radionuclide formulation	**β^- energy (MeV)/ γ energy (keV)**	**Shunt study**
Yttrium-90 (SIR Spheres; TheraSphere)	2.2/-	^{99m}Tc-MAA
Holmium-166 Microspheres	1.84/81	^{99m}Tc-MAA
Iodine-131 Lipiodol	0.606/364	Iodine-131 Lipiodol (Scout dose)
Rhenium-188 Lipiodol	2.12/155	Rhenium-188 Lipiodol (Scout dose)
Rhenium-188 Microspheres	2.12/155	^{99m}Tc-microspheres

Indications:

- Unresectable HCC with or without portal vein thrombosis.
- Small tumor located near a large blood vessel.
- Patient not fit for surgery.
- Neoadjuvant therapy before resection/transplantation.
- Isolated liver metastasis from neuroendocrine, bladder and colorectal cancers.

Eligibility Criteria:

- Stable haematological parameters: Hb ≥ 8 g/dL; leucocytes ≥ 2000/μL; and platelets ≥ 70000/μL.
- Adequate liver function: Bilirubin < 3.0 mg/dL; Albumin ≥ 3.0 g/dL.
- Shunt study for estimation of dose to lungs (should be less than 20 Gy to avoid radiation pneumonitis), normal liver (should be < 30 Gy to prevent liver damage) and bowel (to avoid ulcers).
- Patients with ascites or other liver failure signs, pregnancy, uncontrolled coagulopathy, and unsafe vascular access to the lesion are excluded.

Treatment Protocol:

- Stop kinase inhibitor drugs like sorafenib ten days prior to therapy.
- Pre-therapy assessments: clinical history, laboratory tests (complete blood counts, serum creatinine, prothrombin time, AST, ALT, alkaline phosphatase), serology for hepatitis B or C infection) Child's score, alpha-fetoprotein (AFP) and portal vein status.
- Triple phase (TP) CT, MRI or PET with TPCT for treatment planning.
- Written and informed consent from the patient.
- The catheter is placed via femoral artery puncture by an interventional radiologist in the Digital Subtraction Angiography (DSA) room.
- Deliver scout dose of 3-5 mCi (111-185 MBq) of Tc-99m MAA or same formulation used for SIRT.
- Whole body image is acquired under gamma camera equipped with a suitable collimator for shunt study in the Nuclear Medicine department.
- Regional SPECT/CT is more suitable for lung shunt (% ratio of lung and lung+liver counts) and calculation of dose to normal liver (tumour to normal liver ratio).
- The patient is shifted back to DSA and therapy dose is delivered.

- Post therapy image is acquired after 24 hours, and the patient is discharged.
- The response is assessed using changes in tumour size and enhancement (modified RECIST criteria) at 2-3 months post therapy with TPCT or PET/TPCT.

Efficacy and Toxicity:

- Overall survival of patients treated with SIRT does not differ from patients treated with trans-arterial chemo-embolization (TACE).
- SIRT is better tolerated and demonstrates improved quality of life.

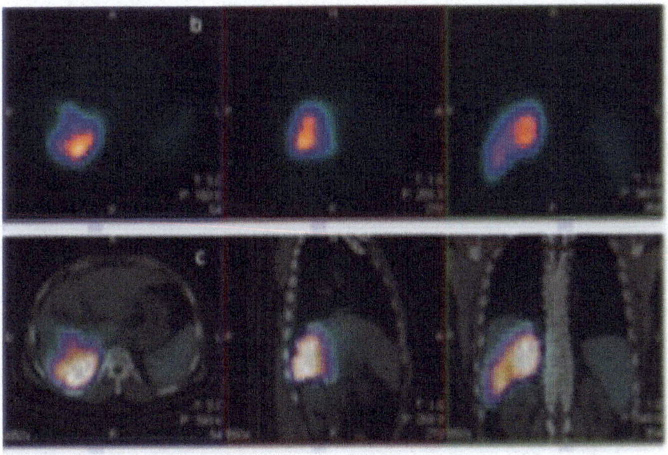

*A 48 years male with chronic liver disease with enhancing lesion in segment VI-VII of liver (6.5*8.8 cm) and portal vein thrombosis (AFP: 213 ng/ml). Patient was treated with 150 mCi ^{188}Re-Microspheres SIRT.*

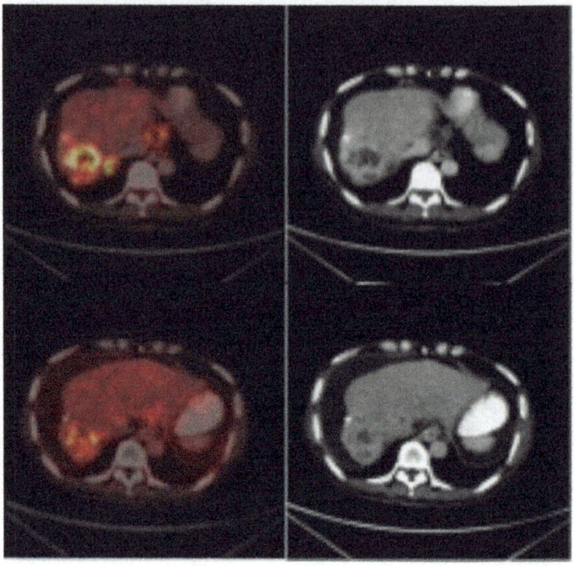

Pre-therapy ^{18}*F-FDG PET/CT*

Post-therapy ^{18}*F-FDG PET/CT done after 3 months showing partial response to SIRT*

11.7 Radiosynovectomy

- Radiosynovectomy (RSV) is a local form of radionuclide therapy for inflamed joints.
- RSV is useful for the treatment of refractory synovitis after failure of drug therapy and intra-articular steroid injections.
- After intra-articular injection, the radiopharmaceutical colloidal particles are phagocytosed by macrophages in the inflamed synovium, and beta particles cause ablation of inflamed synovial membrane and fibrosis.

Radiopharmaceuticals	Physical decay	Half-life (days)
^{90}Y-citrate/silicate	β^-	2.7
^{186}Re-sulfide	β^-, γ	3.7
^{188}Re-tin colloid	β^-, γ	0.7
^{169}Er-citrate	β^-	9.45

β^-, Beta; γ, Gamma

Indications:

- Inflammatory joint disorders;
  - Rheumatoid arthritis,
  - Spondylarthropathy (e.g. reactive or psoriatic arthritis),
  - Lyme disease/Behcet´s disease.

- Calcium pyrophosphate dihydrate (CPPD) arthritis,
- Pigmented villonodular synovitis (PVNS),
- Undifferentiated arthritis,
- Haemophilic arthritis,
- Osteoarthritis with active inflammation.

Contraindications: Local skin infection, hemarthrosis, or ruptured popliteal cyst around knee. Pregnancy and lactation are general contraindications.

Eligibility criteria: Painful swollen joint with synovitis refractory to intra-articular steroids.

Treatment protocol:

- For knee, exclude a ruptured Baker's cyst or hemarthrosis. Review MRI of the joint.
- Three-phase ^{99m}Tc-MDP skeletal scintigraphy to assess the severity of active soft-tissue inflammation of the involved joint.
- The minimum time interval between last therapy and RSV:
    - Arthroscopy or joint surgery -6 weeks.
    - Last joint puncture - 2 weeks.
- Informed written consent must be obtained from the patient.
- Dose depends on size of the joint:

Joint	Dose/activity	Injected volume
Large joints (Hip/knee/shoulder)	12-20 mCi (444-740 MBq)	3 ml
Medium joints (Elbow/wrists/ankle)	8-10 mCi (296-370 MBq)	1-1.5 ml
Small joints	0.5-1 mCi (18.5-37 MBq)	1 ml

- The intra-articular injection is done under strict aseptic precautions. Syringe should be flushed with normal saline post-radiotracer administration.
- Patient is instructed tomove the joint for homogenous tracer distribution within the joint after injection.
- The joint needs to be immobilized with a splint for 48 hours, followed by limited physical activity for 1 week.
- After48 hours, post-therapy imaging is done to confirm the tracer distribution in the joint.
- Retreatment can be done after 3 months.

Therapeutic efficacy:

- Overall, 40-90 % success rate for different joints and diseases.
- The response may be delayed for 2-4 weeks after injection.

• 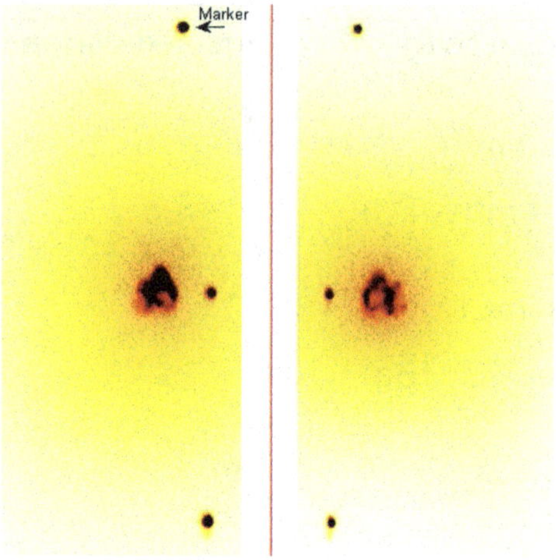

Left knee PVNS post-treatment (with ^{188}Re tin colloid) images.

Adverse effects:

Early: Radiation induced synovitis (transient).

Late: Radiation necrosis (rare).

11.8 Skin Patch Radionuclide Therapy

Skin cancer:

- Skin is exposed to atmospheric Ultraviolet (UV-A and B) radiation.
- UV-B is responsible for non-melanoma skin cancers: basal cell carcinoma (BCC) and squamous cell carcinoma (SCC).
- Artificial sources of sunlight may also cause skin cancer.
- SCC is often metastatic at presentation. BCC is usually non-metastatic, but can be life-threatening when metastatic. Surgical excision is the preferred treatment for localised disease.

Keloid:

- Keloids are fibrotic scars that can develop during the wound healing process at the site of surgery or trauma.
- They often grow beyond the scar and can cause pain and pruritus.
- Surgery is not preferred for keloid as the risk of recurrence is high.
- Keloids can develop at multiple sites all over the body.

Indication for skin Patch Radionuclide Therapy:

- Unresectable skin cancers and keloid can be treated non-invasively with radionuclide skin patch therapy.

Radionuclides	β^- energy (MeV)	Half-life	Tissue penetration
Yttrium-90	2.2	64 hours	11 mm
Holmium-166	1.84	26.8 hours	8.7 mm
Phosphorus-32	1.71	14.3 days	8 mm
Lutetium-177	0.497	6.6 days	1.7 mm
Rhenium-188	2.12	16.9 hours	11 mm

Patch Preparation:

- A trace of the lesion is taken on paper, and the same shape is drawn and cut on an absorbent sheet to prepare a customized patch.
- The area of the lesion is calculated using graph paper.
- Radionuclide activity is uniformly spread on customized patch.
- Patch is dried and laminated using thin and transparent adhesive tape and applied to the lesion.

Treatment Procedure:

- Treatment may be given as fractionated doses or as a single dose.
- Dose delivered is mainly dependent on the energy of radionuclide, physical decay and application time (penetration length and stopping power are also important).
- Fractionated dose regime requires few sittings (2-3) and followed when high-energy long-lived radionuclide is used.

- Skin carcinoma and mature keloids are treated with high radiation absorbed dose (100 Gy).

- Newly formed keloids are treated with lower radiation absorbed dose (50-75 Gy).

Advantages:

- Tailor-made radioactive patch therapy is a non-invasive outpatient procedure for skin cancer and keloid.

- The maximum dose is deposited within the penetration depth of radionuclide. No systemic side effect and negligible radiation exposure to non-target organs.

- Irradiation dose and time may be individualized.

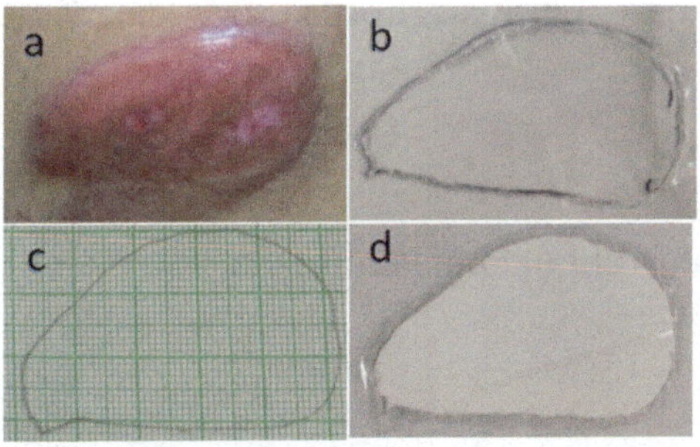

a) Lesion
b) Trace
c) Area calculation
d) Radioactive patch

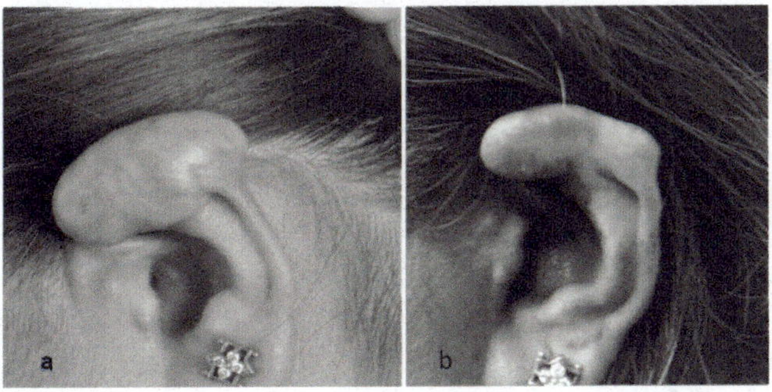

a) Pretherapy keloid of ear
b) Post-therapy reduction in size of the lesion is noted.

11.9 ^{131}I-MIBG Therapy

^{131}I-MIBG radionuclide therapy is an effective treatment option for metastatic neural crest/chromaffin cell tumours.

Radiopharmaceutical	Physical decay (Energy)	Half-life
^{131}I MIBG	β^-(0.606 MeV) γ (0.364 MeV)	8.02 days

β^-, Beta; γ, Gamma

Indications:

- Metastatic pheochromocytoma, paraganglioma or carcinoid tumours.
- Neuroblastoma (Stage III/IV).
- Medullary thyroid cancer (Recurrent or metastatic).

Contraindications:

- Life expectancy less than 3 months.
- Impaired renal function (GFR <30 ml/min).
- Pregnancy and lactation are general contraindications.

Eligibility criteria:

- Treatment refractory progressive metastatic tumours mentioned above (after surgery, radiofrequency ablation, or embolization).

- High tracer uptake on I-123/I-131MIBG scan (2-3 times background uptake in most lesions, *see section 2.4*).
- Haemoglobin >9gm/dL, TLC >3,500/mm^3 and platelets >10^5/mm^3 within 1 week.
- Bilirubin and liver enzymes < 2 times of the normal values;
- Drugs that interfere with MIBG uptake should be withdrawn before therapy.

Treatment protocol:

- The thyroid gland can take up free radioiodine in MIBG preparation. It should be blocked by giving oral stable iodine 48 hours before therapy and 7–14 days post-therapy;
- Prophylactic antiemetic to be given before infusion;
- Slow intravenous infusion (over 1to 3 hours) via cannula or central venous line using a shielded infusion system;
- ^{131}I-MIBG Dose: 100-300 mCi (3.7-11.1 GBq)/therapy cycle;
- Vitals should be checked during treatment infusion and at least twice daily afterwards. Alpha or beta-blockers may be required in the event of catecholamine release from tumour destruction.

Therapeutic efficacy: 30-47% in pheochromocytoma and paraganglioma, 30% in neuroblastoma and medullary thyroid cancer.

Adverse effects:

Early: Transient hypertension during infusion, nausea and vomiting.

Late: Marrow suppression, renal dysfunction and hypothyroidism (in case of insufficient thyroid blockade).

Bibliography & Suggested Reading

1. O'Malley JP, Ziessman HA, & Thrall JH. Nuclear Medicine and Molecular Imaging: The Requisites, 5th Edition(2020). Philadelphia: Elsevier.
2. Cherry SR, Sorenson JA, & Phelps ME. Physics in Nuclear Medicine, 4th Edition (2012). Philadelphia: Saunders.
3. Society of Nuclear Medicine and Molecular Imaging (SNMMI) Procedure Standards (https://www.snmmi.org).
4. European Association of Nuclear Medicine (EANM) Guidelines (https://www.eanm.org/publications/guidelines).
5. European Nuclear Medicine Guide (https://www.nucmed-guide.app).
6. National Comprehensive Cancer Network Clinical Practice Guidelines in Oncology (NCCN Guidelines®) (https://www.nccn.org/guidelines).
7. American thyroid association (ATA) guidelines (https://www.thyroid.org/professionals/ata-professional-guidelines/)
8. Nuclear Medicine Journals:
    a. Seminars in Nuclear Medicine
    b. Journal of Nuclear Medicine (JNM)
    c. Journal of Nuclear Cardiology (JNC)
    d. IndianJournal of Nuclear Medicine (IJNM)

Appendix

Effective radiation dose from Nuclear Medicine procedures

Radiopharmaceutical	Dose coefficient (mSv/mCi)*	Administered activity (in mCi,adults)	Effective dose (mSv)
^{99m}Tc-Pertechnetate	0.481	5	2.4
^{99m}Tc-Sestamibi	0.314	20	6.28
^{99m}Tc-MDP	0.296	20	5.92
^{99m}Tc-DTPA	0.181	5	0.91
^{99m}Tc-EC	0.233	5	1.16
^{99m}Tc-MAG3	0.259	5	1.29
^{99m}Tc-DMSA	0.326	3	0.98
^{99m}Tc-Mebrofenin	0.629	4	2.52
^{99m}Tc-RBC	0.259	20	5.18
^{99m}Tc-Tetrofosmin	0.255	30	7.66
^{201}Tl-Chloride	5.18	3	15.54
^{99m}Tc-MAA	0.407	5	2.03
^{99m}Tc-ECD	0.285	20	5.7
^{18}F-DOPA	0.925	5	4.62
^{18}F-FDG	0.703	10	7.03
^{68}Ga-PSMA	0.814	3	2.44
^{68}Ga-DOTATATE	0.777	3	2.33

mSv, milli Sievert; mCi, milli curie. Pediatric dosage will be reduced in proportion to reduction in administered activity. For hybrid PET-CT/SPECT-CT, CT dose will be extra (depending on the CT protocol).

*Adapted from 1. Mattsson S, Johansson L, Liniecki J, et al. Radiation dose to patients from radiopharmaceuticals. World Congress on Medical Physics and Biomedical Engineering. September 2009, Munich, Germany. 474-477.

2. Weber DA, Makler PT Jr, Watson EE, Coffey JL, Thomas SR, London J. MIRD dose estimate report no. 13: radiation absorbed dose from technetium-99m-labeled bone imaging agents. J Nucl Med. 1989;30:1117–1122.

Feedback

We'd love to hear what you think about the book.
Write a review or email us at

nuclearmedicineaprimer@gmail.com

Made in the USA
Las Vegas, NV
26 October 2022

58184106R00109